ADVANCE PRAISE FOR *MAKE LOVE 365 TIMES A YEAR: 7 Sex Secrets for a Passionate Love Life*

"*Make Love 365 Times a Year: 7 Sex Secrets for a Passionate Love Life* is a must-read for any couple wanting to keep their relationship alive, exciting, and sexually satisfying. Her use of analogies is great. I especially enjoyed the visual of undealt with feelings and resentment being like a fish stuffed in a drawer, becoming more and more stinky! And her analogies of relationships to cars, the Three-Floor House and Stairway.

I wrote about *the Health Benefits of Sex* in my doctorate and was especially drawn to Dr. Heinz's differentiation between sex and lovemaking. It made me reassess my approach to my own work with couples, and I will recommend her book as a textbook for couples I am working with and encourage *Making Love 365 days a year*!

I can feel Dr. Heinz's passion within her words and the enjoyment she has taken writing this book. It is very detailed and well researched with a lot of her own personal insight and inspiration from years of working with couples, and her life path.

This book is more geared towards heterosexual coupling. Still, there are plenty of gems for us all, whether you are in a relationship with just yourself, in a polyamorous/open relationship, or a same-sex one, if you can read beyond the genderfication and male/female stereotypes."

—Dr. Shelley, sexologist and author of *Anti-Aging & Health Benefits of Sex*

MAKE LOVE
365 TIMES
a YEAR

7 Sex Secrets
FOR A PASSIONATE LOVE LIFE

Aleida Heinz, Ph.D.

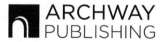
ARCHWAY
PUBLISHING

Archway Publishing books may be ordered through booksellers or by contacting:

Archway Publishing
1663 Liberty Drive
Bloomington, IN 47403
www.archwaypublishing.com
1 (888) 242-5904

Because of the dynamic nature of the Internet, any web addresses or links contained in
this book may have changed since publication and may no longer be valid. The views
expressed in this work are solely those of the author and do not necessarily reflect the
views of the publisher, and the publisher hereby disclaims any responsibility for them.

Any people depicted in stock imagery provided by Getty Images are models,
and such images are being used for illustrative purposes only.
Certain stock imagery © Getty Images.

ISBN: 978-1-4808-9025-1 (sc)
ISBN: 978-1-4808-9024-4 (e)

Library of Congress Control Number: 2020911290

Print information available on the last page.

Archway Publishing rev. date: 6/29/2020

For Pedro, thank you my love, not only for your support but also because it's with you that I live what I preach in this book. For my three wonderful adult-children: Leo, Alejandro, and Patty, who have always been my inspiration.
and
for anyone who wants to make love 365 times a year.

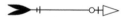

Anyone who is in love is making love the whole time, even
when they're not. When two bodies meet, it is just the cup
overflowing. They can stay together for hours, even days.
They begin the dance one day and finish it the next, or–such
is the pleasure they experience–they may never finish it.

—Paulo Coelho

CONTENTS

SEX SECRET #1

SEX SECRET #2

SEX SECRET #3

SEX SECRET #4

SEX SECRET #5

SEX SECRET #6

SEX SECRET #7

FOREWORD
by Dr. Eusebio Rubio-Aurioles, MD, PhD

A shadow of mystery and secrecy surrounds sexuality. For most of us, educated in the western world, natural sexual curiosity frequently results in guilt, a sense of wrongdoing, and transgression. In contrast, cultural messages include a demand to become sexual experts in our "careers" as sexual partners, life partners, marital prospects, and family pillars.

Have you ever wondered why there are so much mystery and secrecy about our sexuality? The most common experience in growing up in our western cultures is that attempting to learn, understand, let alone beginning to live what sexuality and sexuality-related experiences are all about is accompanied by strongly ambivalent feelings. This reality is in sharp contrast with the portrait of sex, use of sexuality to attain other goals such as marketing effectively a product or merely profiting, that is so commonly seen in the public discourse and media.

In my opinion, this highly explosive cocktail results from a combination of significant degrees of sexual ignorance and a series of culturally validated oversimplifications of what is needed to have a fulfilling and lasting sexual partnership. It should not surprise us that many individuals and couples end up "lost in the woods," to use a metaphor. When one is lost in unknown terrain, what is most needed is a map with precise instructions to get where we really want to go.

Dr. Aleida Heinz has produced exactly what is needed in today's confusing world of demands and anxieties about our sexual potential. In essence, a road map to a very desirable goal: *make love 365 times a year.* Presented as the unveiling of seven sexual secrets, a clear path to develop a fulfilling, gratifying, and lasting lovemaking partnership is offered in a text full of examples, clarity, and precise recommendations.

But writing a book on sexual secrets prompts the expectations in the eventual reader, and many times the one who writes, of a "manual of sex." As if figuring out the repertory of techniques was a real solution to achieve sexual fulfillment. I call this "the magic spot touch approach." Proclaiming that a certain anatomical mystery has been discovered and reaching that spot is a guarantee of sexual satisfaction is both a monument to innocence and ignorance. Been acquainted with the possibilities of our bodies is, of course, essential for the pursuit of sexual pleasure, but attributing almost magical properties to any particular area of the body is misleading.

Thus, knowing our body, its potentials to produce pleasure, and clues for the erotic experience is in fact critical, but, as Dr. Heinz rightfully warns us, the foundations for a fulfilling experience of *making love 365 times a year* lies elsewhere. Building a life with a partner with the possibility of *making love 365 times a year* demands a good foundation, not spectacular adornments that lack a well-grounded basis.

The series of sex secrets described, exemplified and illustrated with ingenious figures, begin with the foundation, what really functions as the basis for the rest of strategies and can be easily summarized by the title *A Sexual Mindset* than translates into an informed, accepting and understanding frame of mind on sexuality. Then a series of practical yet critically essential components of sexual wellbeing: healthy lifestyle, loving feelings, expressing capabilities, pleasure abilities, eroticism, and finally, sexual techniques.

Eroticism has been the focus of my professional life for many years. Interestingly I realized some time ago that in some areas of the world, the term is more related to pornography than to art. Eroticism is the sexual aspect that is more specific to humans, despite some considerations that find the erotic close to our animal nature. As Dr. Heinz correctly explains, our erotic dimension allows for anticipation. Our mindset, knowledge, attitudes, level of acquaintance with our body—especially in its arousal and orgasmic capabilities—conflate at particular moments in life to anticipate. I cannot refrain from citing one of the most erotic scenes in the cinema: the 1993 movie *The Piano* directed by Jane Campion. The scene where the first physical contact between the two lovers occurs with the tip of the finger that touches the narrow hole, left by a torn stocking, which allows direct contact with the leg. The film correctly portrays the intensity that anticipation can produce.

What you have in your hands is a truly useful tool. The clarity and extensive use of examples taken directly from Dr. Heinz's clinical practice has produced a very effective roadmap. I congratulate Dr. Heinz for this effort and urge the reader to take practical steps clearly suggested in the text to continue the effort to build a relationship, first with yourself and then, when the time comes, with your partner, correct courses or start the journey from the beginning. The benefits of having a fulfilling sexual life are clear nowadays, let's work towards this and let's live a more fulfilling life.

Dr. Eusebio Rubio-Aurioles, MD, PhD
Past President of the World Association for Sexual Health (WAS).
First President of the Federación Mexicana de Educación Sexual y Sexología, A.C.
Founder and General Director at Asociación Mexicana para
la Salud Sexual, A.C. (Amssac) Amssac.org

ACKNOWLEDGMENTS

What prompted me to carry out this great project of writing a non-fiction book? The initial idea to write something, be it a book, a text, a program for couples, etc., came from my oldest son Leonardo (Leo) long ago. Since then, the idea of writing has remained in my mind. But write about what? I could write about infidelity, how to seduce a man or a woman, how to be a better partner, better sex, or many other inexhaustible topics.

Upon my arrival in the United States, I began writing newspaper and magazine articles in English and Spanish. I started to truly like the idea of writing, always motivated by my dear husband Pedro, whom I thank infinitely for all his support. His love and his total confidence in my professional ability motivated me to continue writing. We even wrote a book together: *The In-Factor: How the Internet Leads to Infidelity*, and ever since, I started writing only in English, which was a big challenge for me. I made the final decision to write a book during a Tony Robbins event in New Jersey in 2015, exactly one year after our house burned down. During the event, I said to myself: YES! I can do it, and I will do it. That is where my journey and my challenge began.

After ideas, thousands of notes, essays, and even dreams, I was able to formulate and elaborate on the message that I wanted to transmit to all people, especially to all couples around the world. I thank my friend JoAnne Shields for her invaluable help with grammar and her encouragement. To my son Leo, who spent time and energy understanding my graphics and turning them into real digital images and illustrations. I thank my development editor Jennifer Blanchard for her wonderful work. To all my clients who took the Lovemaking Wheel. To Dr. Eusebio Rubio-Aurioles for writing such a beautiful foreword for my book. Eternally grateful to my parents, who always believed in me, especially my father, who passed away in 2012 and who would be very proud of this work.

To the love and support of my other children Alejandro (Ale) and Patricia (Patty). Once again to Pedro, "mi papi," whom I love so much and with whom I *make love 365 times a year.* And to all my family, friends, clients, and people around me who have been enthusiastic about this book.

Thank you!

INTRODUCTION

There is abundant scientific evidence supporting the multiple benefits of having healthy sex. Improving your love life will have a tremendous positive impact on your overall mental and physical well-being and, of course, on your relationship satisfaction. Sex is about "me," love is about "you," and lovemaking is about "us." This book is about "us"—you and your partner or future partner—learning to *make love 365 times a year*, with me guiding you. *Making love 365 times a year* can transform your entire relationship, bring your connection to an even deeper level, and change your life!

Lovemaking is a beautiful, healthy, and sustainable activity you can enjoy over and over. I have found that lovemaking is the key to keeping any relationship healthy, passionate, fulfilling, and enjoyable. Relationship satisfaction is crucial for your sex life, and your sex life is essential for a happy and healthy relationship. Therefore, your relationship and your sex life go hand-in-hand, and both determine the quality of your love life. By strengthening your love life, you will improve your life experience in general, but to accomplish this, you must work on yourself first.

I often hear that it is easier to remain sexually passive and do nothing than it is to work on building passion. People have frequently asked me if it's possible to have great sex every day. While I do not think it's possible, making love every day is. Surely you can make love every day. Therefore, my answer is always: why not? Find out for yourself, unlock your sexual potential, and learn the art of lovemaking now! It is never too late!

What do you need to unlock the potential to *make love 365 times a year*? The energy, some knowledge, intention, strategy, action, and most importantly: LOVE. Knowledge is information. The aim, work, along with accurate information, determine your power to create a delightful love life and to *make love 365 times a year.*

Make Love 365 Times a Year: 7 Sex Secrets for a Passionate Love Life is not just a book about sex. Sex and lovemaking are two different acts, with two different purposes. Lovemaking goes beyond sexual techniques and orgasm; it involves love as well as many other variables. This project is an attempt to help you sustain a healthy and passionate love life and to remain connected to your partner throughout time. I am not suggesting in any way that you have risky, irresponsible, or non-consensual sex. I am talking about lovemaking: always loving, consensual, responsible, safe, and pleasurable.

Connectivity, which keeps a couple happily together, and the elements to sustain it, are the basis of my work. I intend to offer you a new and fresh way to view sex: a more sophisticated approach that allows you to make love every day, for as long as you want, until the end of your life, to stay connected to your partner, and, at the same time, grow as individuals.

Make Love 365 Times a Year: 7 Sex Secrets for a Passionate Love Life is an ideal book for you if you want a satisfying, passionate, and long-lasting love life. This book is a guide for adults of any age, sexual orientation, race, or culture, in a closed or open relationship who want to build and maintain a passionate love life. This book focuses mostly on how to do it, rather than discussing why it's essential to have healthy sex.

For those men, women, and couples who want to make love or want to make more love: I firmly believe that lovemaking is the ultimate connection to total sexual pleasure and the cornerstone of passionate relationships. Being strongly connected will allow you to make love continuously and vice-versa. It is a never-ending circle of joy and love.

For twenty years, I have been searching to find out why most couples in long-term relationships refuse the privilege of experiencing—or sometimes even thinking about—something as beautiful as lovemaking. The truth is that only a few long-term committed couples have a love life full of passion. Why?

Most couples enter into marriage, wanting to enjoy a long-lasting life of sexual intimacy and satisfaction. Yet, statistics show that over 60%—I think even more—of married couples no longer have satisfying, or even existent, sexual relationships with their partners. The result? Divorce, infidelity, loneliness, or the so-called "roommate couples" or "sexless relationships." As a couple counselor and board-certified sexologist, I can certainly attest to this number. For the past twenty years, I have counseled, mentored, and helped thousands of "sexless couples" to overcome the hurt and bleakness of passionless relationships.

Americans are now having less sex than ever before, not to mention less lovemaking. A recent article in the Achieves of Sexual Behavior shows that married couples in America are losing their passion and are having sex nine times less per year than they were in the 1990s. People now believe that this lack of sex, in long-term relationships, is typical, because our society portrays it as such. Many people, movies and television shows treat the lack of sex in long-term committed relationships as "normal."

As couples begin to have children or build a life together, they often become complacent and no longer expect sexual passion in their relationship, making it "a stage" or "phase." Every day in my practice, I help frustrated couples change such beliefs and update their mindsets about lovemaking. To some, this decline seems inevitable, but I know it is not!

I have found that dissatisfied couples share specific characteristics—variables—that prevent them from enjoying their sex life in healthy ways. These couples do not know what they need to work on to improve their love life. So, I have classified these variables into seven different areas, which I call the *7 Sex Secrets*. In this way, individuals and couples can identify what their problems are and begin to work on them. These seven variables are the foundation of this book.

There does not exist a magic formula or "pill" for lovemaking. There's not just one, or two, things that you or your partner must do to experience this kind of bliss. A combination of critical elements—the *7 Sex Secrets*—plus continuous effort, will give you the possibility of an ideal love life.

Make Love 365 Times a Year: 7 Sex Secrets for a Passionate Love Life comes from my clinical observations and findings after years of experience guiding couples to improve their love lives. My research goes from what these couples lack to what they need. This book is not based on a survey; instead, the information and material comes from my 20+ years of experience in private practice: from my sessions with couples, my academic studies, research from excellent specialists, and my own experience as a woman, wife, and lover. I work with all kinds of couples, some distant and some nearby, in both English and Spanish.

Make Love 365 Time a Year: 7 Sex Secrets for a Passionate Love Life comprises seven chapters—the *7 Sex Secrets*. Each chapter is a "Sex Secret," arranged in order of importance. Don't get me wrong—I don't mean to say that the last chapter is not important or that only the first ones are essential. Each chapter is important and contains five parts, and, also includes suggestions and book references. It is best to read the chapters consecutively since the first Sex Secret is the most important and each one builds upon the others, but you can start with any chapter you want if your goal is to improve a specific area in your love life.

Make Love 365 Time a Year: 7 Sex Secrets for a Passionate Love Life also includes a unique tool I have created: *The Lovemaking Wheel*, a chart which serves to help you identify and evaluate your lovemaking behavior. You can track your progress in each area of lovemaking, ultimately revealing both your strongest and weakest points. Central to the Lovemaking Wheel is a short questionnaire that deals with the seven aspects of lovemaking—sexual attitudes, health, emotions, feelings, sexual abilities, eroticism, and the capacity to explore pleasure and to communicate.

You will place a dot in each section based on your answers from the questionnaire. Dots closer to the center show there is room for work; dots closer to the outside show that area is doing great. You and your partner can then connect the dots to see the shape of your Lovemaking Wheel—found in the Appendix. The bigger the wheels, the better your connection and the possibilities for endless lovemaking. Ideally, you and your partner's Lovemaking Wheels will eventually overlap.

Case studies are a powerful way to share what I want you to know in each chapter in order to do the work. Therefore, I have selected real-life-cases of couples I've worked with who were dealing with a specific problem in each of the seven areas. I have chosen heterosexual couples of different ages and cultures, in closed relationships, because they represent most of my cases. The names and specific details of my clients were changed to protect their identities and privacy.

At the beginning of each chapter, I describe a client case illustrating a specific problem of how the couple was affected. I see variations of these cases over and over; each case is different, though certain problem areas that I have identified are common to all of them. I have also included the Lovemaking Wheels for these seven couples, to show you their weakest points and how it affected their sex lives. So, you will find a total of 14 Lovemaking Wheels—one per person, two per chapter—throughout the book. I invite you to do one of your own!

I will explain to you some of the work I did with my case-study clients, and what I suggested precisely as far as activities, exercises, and advice for making these changes. Most people cannot work on their problems by themselves; therefore, some guidance is always necessary. That is the purpose of this book.

In this book, you will find original and innovative models I have crafted, such as The *LOVEX* Model (Chapter 3), The *Infidelity-Fidelity* Model (Chapter 3), The *Three-Floor House* (Chapter 4), The *Pleasure Spectrum* Model (Chapter 5), and *Eroticism: The Stairway to Sexual Pleasure* (Chapter 6). These new models explain and illustrate the different concepts that I work with my clients on.

In my opinion, there is nothing more fulfilling for your life than a healthy relationship with passion, that allows you to be connected to your partner and to experience lovemaking as part of your existence. Think well and choose right, then do the work! Renowned anthropologist Helen Fisher, PhD, has proclaimed "we are born to love." So, love and do not be afraid to make love! As cardiologist Dr. Steven Gundry, MD, says, "what good is a long, healthy life if you can't spend it with the people you love? Human connection really seems to drive successful aging—not to mention the motivation to stay alive and vibrant."

It is possible to have sex without passion, but it will not last. Passion implies a warm and constant emotion towards your partner, with whom you'll share an eager interest and an energetic pursuit to make love. Any man, any woman, any couple can learn the *7 Sex Secrets* to *make love 365 times a year* with passion, devotion, and endurance, and to stay happily together throughout the years.

From my earliest days in Rio de Janeiro, I have always had a passion for life. To me, Brazil seemed like a magical world full of passion and love, where anything was possible. As a young girl, I began to look at the relationships that surrounded me, most notably that of my parents. Everywhere I looked, I saw happy, passionate couples. Passion is what I wanted in my own life. Now you can have it in yours, too!

My professional passion has always been to understand and express what it means for couples to be intimate and passionate, and to express their love in the best possible way. I believed there had to be a way to keep the passion alive and it was my deepest wish to find out how.

Now, I want to share in this book what I have learned and experienced—not just in my years of private practice, but also in my personal life. I hope this book will encourage you to *make love 365 times a year* and enjoy it! To love and be loved is what our souls need. Fisher once said, "a world without love is a deadly place." For me, a romantic relationship without lovemaking is a dead relationship.

I hope all couples will learn the 7 key elements to unlock sexual potential and make love every day, as the ultimate way to keep the connection as romantic partners. It is a precious thing! If you do not have a partner now, you can still learn from this book and be ready for when you do. The decision to choose a partner is one of the most—if not the most—important decisions of your life; it can take you to heaven or hell; it can bring out the best in you when it's healthy, or it can make you miserable and lonely when it's dysfunctional.

I wrote *Make Love 365 Times a Year: 7 Sex Secrets for a Passionate Love Life* with a lot of love and dedication. With my twenty years of professional experience, I can reassure you that building and maintaining a happy, healthy, and fulfilling relationship full of passion is possible. It is also possible to *make love 365 times a year*, and the effort you put in will lead to a strong, deep connection with your partner.

I hope you take what you learn from this book and use it so you and your partner, or future partner, can be sexually happy and satisfied for the rest of your lives.

Now, enjoy the book, enjoy your partner—or find the right partner first—and then *make love 365 times a year* to stay deeply connected. You can make it happen. Open your minds and your hearts to take this new journey together!

Aleida Heinz, PhD, Charlotte, NC, 2020

SEX SECRET

CHAPTER 1

A Sexual Mindset

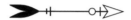

> Sex lies at the root of life, and we can never learn to
> reverence life until we know how to understand sex.
> —Havelock Ellis

Part I: The Power of Your Mind

Your mind has a great, unbelievable power; a power that is not yet fully understood by science. As you may see in the following client case, individuals who hold false, outdated, and negative beliefs about sex have problems experiencing satisfaction in their love lives. As world-renowned Stanford University psychologist Carol S. Dweck, PhD, says, "beliefs are the key to happiness and to misery." Psychologist David Schnarch, PhD, also shares the same view that "the beliefs and practices we share with many couples are the sources of our misery." It is very important that you and your partner become aware of your beliefs about sex, sexuality, love, and romantic relationships. Having outdated beliefs can negatively impact your sex life.

As Dweck explains, negative beliefs cause negative feelings in all aspects of our lives. "Our minds are constantly monitoring and interpreting," she says. "But sometimes the interpretation process goes awry." Dweck believes that "you can change your mindset; it's about stretching yourself to learn something new. Developing yourself." This chapter is about showing you how important your mindset about sexuality is for an active sex life, how necessary it is to work and improve your mindset, and how to do so in order to enjoy a healthy relationship and *make love 365 times a year.*

In the following client case, the beliefs, attitudes, and expectations of this couple toward sex and sexuality were very negative, causing sexual avoidance, false expectations, and dissatisfaction. Even though the male partner had a somewhat better attitude toward sex than the female, he was suffering as well. This can mean that if your partner has negative beliefs and attitudes toward sex, you can have them too and suffer as well. Let's see this fact with our first case. The following statements were taken from my notes in sessions with these clients.

Case #1: Eli & Chris

Married couple Elizabeth and Christian (Eli and Chris), ages 35 and 37 years old respectively; married for five years, and no children.

When Eli and Chris first came to my practice, I asked them what brought them to me.

"Lack of…intimacy," Eli first said.

"Intimacy issues," Chris agreed.

People usually do not have a clear understanding of what intimacy is—which means intercourse for them—and often confuse it with sex. Intimacy is about disclosing ourselves, and sex is what we *do* with our genitals—sexual activities. I will address intimacy and sex in other chapters. So, Eli and Chris were trying to communicate that they were not having sex at all—sexual activities. They, like many people, were confusing sex with intimacy.

In many ways, Eli and Chris seemed to be a perfect couple—both in their early thirties, working full-time, healthy, owned a house, no kids—yet—but they had only been married for five years and were already suffering.

"We're struggling with a lack of physical intimacy." Eli said. "He only wants sex! We've a great relationship—we love each other, but when it comes to sex, we get angry."

According to the couple, when they were dating, they agreed to not have sex (meaning intercourse) due to their religious beliefs. Once married, they found that sex was not what they thought it would be.

"Now that I'm married, I believe that good sex should be natural and spontaneous," Eli explained. "But it's not. It's awkward. It sucks."

Chris quickly took over the conversation. "She has the idea in her head that she's being used just because I wanna have sex with her," he said. "She thinks that having oral is gross and that sex is just for men. She believes that oral sex isn't sex and that it's gross."

Eli did not contradict him as he went on.

"I've always felt guilty about sex because of my religion," she said. "That's why we both agreed on no sex before marriage. Now that we're married, I still feel guilty about sex. We both like each other, love each other a lot, but I feel guilty about initiating, and feel obligated to do it."

Chris replied, "Eli sees it as her wifely duty. It isn't for her pleasure but only to please me. This situation sucks and makes us tense and unhappy. I love her, but I'm tired of this situation."

Chris continued to point at Eli as the source of their problems.

"I'm not using her," he said. "I love her, but she believes sex is another duty, like washing the dishes. Even on our honeymoon she didn't want to do it; she just wanted to be held. We've only had good sex for two days during our whole marriage."

He explained that he bought a book on sex positions, and Eli looked through it. They had fun trying different things for two days before she forgot about the book. Then, she returned to her no-sex attitude.

"She never initiates either," Chris added.

Eli agreed. "I'd like to have a normal and regular sex life, but I just can't," she said. "I never stop thinking negative stuff about sex. I think sex isn't good for me. It's awful. I've never talked about sex with my family or friends."

Eli's mother used to say that sex was for men and was only done to have babies. Talking about it in her household was prohibited. Eli believed that sex would come naturally, but it didn't.

"It scared me," she said. "Now I don't know what to believe. I think it's wrong to have those kinds of thoughts; I don't masturbate, I think that it is wrong too."

Usually, when meeting with clients, I ask the same questions about sex. First: what do you think about sex? What is sex for you? What does sex mean to you? And, what are your expectations?

Eli answered the question quickly. "I believe sex should be about love, and the affection we have for one another," she said. But then—silence.

She thought about the last question a while before answering. "I don't know what it means to me," she said. "It's something I must do as a wife. If he asks me, I'll do it, but it means nothing to me. It isn't important."

Chris answered the questions more confidently.

"To me, sex is a connection," he said. "I'm a pretty good husband. I provide everything for her, including a good home. She should wanna be with me. It's her responsibility to be available when I want her." You can see Chris's outdated beliefs about sex being a marital duty, which makes him expect something not possible from his wife—to enjoy something that she doesn't want to do.

Chris continued, "I want a life together: kids, passion, travel, to be happy. I don't know why this is so difficult for her. She doesn't even wanna talk about sex. I'm not satisfied with our sex; I wanna fix this."

"I always appreciated her, from the beginning, but she's so tense and always avoids me. She doesn't want me to touch her; she limits me. I feel frustrated," he said.

Eli countered, expressing her beliefs and feelings, "I want his support and his tender affection. I want to be a mother, a good wife, to take care of my family, my house, and have a good time together. But I feel angry when he wants sex. I don't have a desire for that; it's gross, and I don't need it. Sex is dirty. And I don't want to have babies right now. I think he's always waiting for sex. He has something in his mind that I don't understand. I don't feel comfortable having sex. I'm too busy and too tired. I feel he only wants me for that reason; that's the only reason he's affectionate. He wants to jack off. That's not loving."

I finished by asking them how they feel now. "I feel confused," Eli said. "I feel frustrated," Chris repeated.

On their Lovemaking Wheels, it is very clear to see that element #1: a sexual mindset—the most important element of all for sexual happiness—is too low. On a scale of 1 to 5, with 5 being the highest, Eli rated too low, rating it at 1. Chris rated it at 2. A sexual mindset was the lowest element for both Eli and Chris, making it very difficult for them to engage in and enjoy their sexuality.

As you will learn, sexual negativity causes sexual avoidance and problems that you may not see. Both Eli and Chris suffered unnecessarily due to their outdated way of thinking about sex, which was affecting both: their intimacy and their sex life.

As the sessions progressed, their willingness to learn and to know more about sex and its benefits increased. They both made great progress, updating their mindsets regarding sexuality and overcoming taboos and false beliefs, in order to believe and accept their sexuality as a healthy part of themselves.

Chris was very patient and supportive of his wife. These days, after a lot of work together, they are enjoying a happy sex life.

They are working on Sex Secret #1: a sexual mindset—the first and foremost ingredient for a happy, satisfactory love life to *make love 365 times a year.*

Please now observe Eli's and Chris's Lovemaking Wheels. See how low Sex Secret #1 is compared to the other aspects or Sex Secrets:

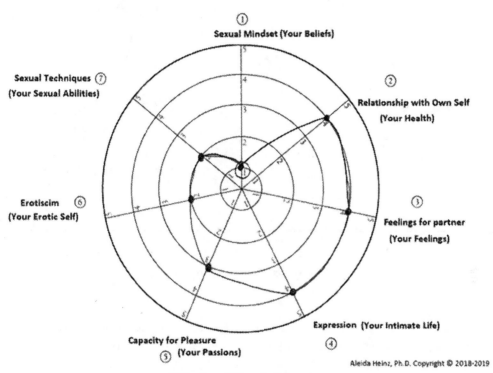

Eli's Sex Wheel -Wheel #1

Aleida Heinz, Ph.D. Copyright © 2018-2019

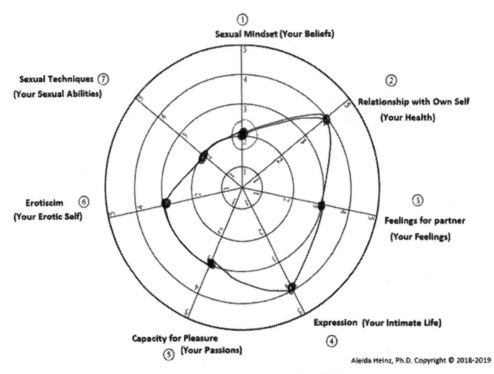

Chris's Sex Wheel -Wheel #2

Willpower and determination are crucial to the process of resetting your mindset about anything—in this case, sex, love, and relationships. For this case study, I started talking about willpower (we will review willpower later in this chapter) and learning to control yourself and your behaviors after both members of the relationship have gathered enough information through scientific evidence, reading recommended books, and doing research about the subject.

I recommended that Eli and Chris, first and foremost, learn more about sexuality outside of their sessions with me, before trying to implement any of the skills learned within the sessions. Knowledge always comes first in order to be aware of why you are doing a certain thing or behaving in a certain way.

After searching for facts, learning, and behaving accordingly to what is learned, the creation of new love habits will eventually emerge. Repetition without knowledge may easily fade, while repetition with understanding will not.

Eli and Chris took the following steps, as I recommend in Part V of this chapter: I first asked them to deeply meditate on the precise messages they were sending to their brains regarding sex, sexuality, relationships, and love in general. Then I encouraged them to ask themselves these questions:

▶ Is this mindset helping me? Do I have a positive sexual mindset? What is my partner's sexual mindset?
▶ Is my mindset taking me to my sexual goals?
▶ Is my sexual mindset logical or reasonable? Are my beliefs rational or irrational?
▶ Why do I think this way? Why do I react this way?
▶ Are my views on sex and relationships the same as my parents, my community, and my religion?
▶ What does sex and sexuality mean to me? To my partner? Are we sexually happy?

That was the first stage. Then, Eli and Chris had to substitute their old negative beliefs with the new positive ones. They had to think about these positive thoughts consciously every day, especially before being sexually together.

You need to truly believe these new positive mindsets first for them to work. Eli and Chris were able to do it and they made it! It takes work, as does every process in life, but it is worth.

My hope is that by reading the following sections or parts, you may understand more about how to modify, enhance, and improve your sexual mindset so you can *make love 365 times a year.*

Part II: Understanding the Inseparable Duo: *Mind & Brain*

One of the most amazing fields for me is Neuroscience. Neuroscience is the scientific study of the brain and the nervous system. The brain is the organ that enables us to learn and adapt to our environment. And, by the way, it is also our main sex organ! Psychology, on the other hand, is the scientific study of the mind: mental functions, human behavior, emotions, and thoughts. The mind has two sides: the unconscious mind—the side we're not aware of, the autopilot, that which houses our core beliefs; and the conscious mind—awareness we have, the pilot, that which houses thoughts and ideas. The mind—in autopilot or pilot—leads the brain in normal conditions.

Neuroplasticity—brain plasticity—which I strongly believe in, is the brain's capacity to be malleable rather than static. Neuroplasticity is the ability of the brain to adapt and change. "Neuro" is for the nerve cells or neurons, and "plastic" refers to the modifiable nature of our brain and nervous system," explains Karen Onderko, Director of Research and Education at Integrated Listening Systems (ILS), a multi-sensory program which integrates music and movement for the purpose of improving emotional regulation, sensory/cognitive processing and motor function.

It means that the brain can reorganize itself, form new neural connections, grow, and improve itself. As Dweck explains in *Mindset*, "new research shows that the brain is more like a muscle—it changes and gets stronger when you use it." Yes! There is enough evidence that our brains grow and get stronger when we learn new things. One way to improve your brain—besides learning new things—is by telling yourself and other people positive stories, and truly believing them. "Neuroscience tells us that a well-told story affects the brain in the same way that actually experiencing the event would," according to Brian Gorman, CPC, in his article *What's the Story*, in *Choice* magazine. He tells us that "when we believe our stories, they often become our truths; sometimes they become our limiting beliefs."

That is, by using the power of your mind to mold your brain, you are growing your brain to work for you, not against you! So, let's first understand a little bit more about this amazing duo: mind and brain, and how they interact. So, consider the brain and mind as two separate and different entities that coexist and exchange information constantly. Your brain is the physical gray structure in your head, like a muscle to be used. Since it is an organ, it can be trained. You can actually see the brain. I call the brain the "chemical factory."

On the other hand, the mind. Your mind is the spiritual and invisible part, so to speak, the non-manifested potential, capable of improving the brain. The mind is the part that flows and guides brain activity. I call the mind the "CEO of the chemical factory." Your mind determines everything you do and how you do it, leading your brain and body to do those actions. The mind controls the brain and "the body does what your brain tells it to do," as described by Dr. Stan Beecham, sports psychologist, leadership consultant, and author of *Elite Minds*.

As neuroscience has proven, your brain will follow for good or bad what you think, tell, or say to yourself. So, always keep in mind that these individual entities—brain and mind—work together as a unit to rule all aspects of your life, including your sexuality.

Even though brain and mind are different entities, they are inseparable. Like a sailboat and wind, the sailboat goes where the wind goes—and your brain goes where your mind goes. You can have a perfectly working sailboat, but with no wind, you have no direction to steer your boat. The wind gives direction to the sailboat. Likewise, your mind gives direction to your brain. Nothing moves until the wind hits the boat…

To fully take advantage of your brain ("your chemical factory"), you must change, improve, modify, and update your mindset—your thoughts, ideas, attitudes, and knowledge, which lead to your expectations, according to your core beliefs. At this point, it is crucial to start evaluating your core beliefs about sex, that may be obsolete and therefore limiting, as explained by Beecham. In *Elite Minds*, Beecham writes that "most of the things we learn and accept as truth take place at the unconscious level. Even if the information is false or inaccurate, it is accepted at the unconscious level as truth…instead of always standing firm in our beliefs, what we should be doing in order to grow is challenging our beliefs."

This is how you think about things and believe in them as if they were truths. So, give yourself permission to challenge your belief system and the way you think about being sexual—regardless of whether you are in a relationship— because there are no changes without challenges! Moreover, there is a common misconception that we only use around 10% of our brain. Dr. Sam Wang, a prominent neuroscientist, professor of Molecular Biology at Princeton University and author of the bestselling book *Welcome to Your Brain*, says that we actually use 100% of our brain—but this wrong idea that we only use 10% of the brain may confuse us.

Be aware that your brain main function is survival. It mainly pays attention to your past to protect you and keep you alive. On the other hand, your mind main function is to find opportunities to grow and learn, therefore, it mainly pays attention to the future, to find ways to improve yourself. Mind by nature is adventurous and fearless. In my opinion, when we are conscious of how mind and brain work, we can be more in the present—not in the past, not in the future—making our minds and brains meeting in the here and now; "calming and nurturing one another." That is why focus (as I will discuss later) is so important; because it makes you stay in the present—you, your mind, and your brain.

Since you know that your brain proceeds according to your thoughts, you must make sure those thoughts are positive, productive, and constructive. You must feed your brain with proper, updated, positive, and correct information for it to grow well and in your favor. It needs a great message to deliver! High brain activity means that your mind is very active, thinking, re-evaluating, imagining, producing, and creating, using 100% of your brain potential.

Brain and mind are an interconnected team. The brain regulates the whole body through the hormones and chemicals it releases. When the brain is confused by receiving wrong messages from the mind or when the brain is unhealthy or damaged, it sends out imbalanced chemicals—aka negative information—leading to negative chemistry. Confusion and negativity may lead to depression, anxiety, and problems in your love life, among other issues. When your brain isn't healthy, it will be very hard to follow the messages your mind is sending it; and most likely your mind isn't healthy either. A healthy brain will always follow the mind, healthy or unhealthy, for good or for bad. A healthy brain is as important as a healthy mind for a happy life and to *make love 365 times a year.*

Studies have shown that continued negative thinking changes a person's brain chemistry for the worse; so, shifting from negative self-talk to positive self-talk is an excellent way towards better brain health. Dr. Richard Carmona, MD, MPH, FACS, one of the leading surgeons in the United States, is an advocate of keeping a healthy brain by avoiding stress, anxiety, and depression. Sounds so simple, but it rarely is…

In her article *Facing Our Patterns*, Janet M. Harvey, MCC, CMC, CCS, wrote that the most effective way towards big and lasting changes is "from the inside out." Harvey explains that "we have the freedom to choose instead of being unconsciously (automatically, autopilot) influenced by limiting beliefs and /or the circumstances in our life." Moreover, Gorman explains that "when we believe our stories, they often become our truths; sometimes they become our limiting beliefs."

Work on both your mind and brain at the same time. Improve your brain by nourishing it properly, drinking plenty of water, thinking, reading, meditating, and having a healthy lifestyle in general. Improve your mind by strengthening it with challenging thinking, updating your mindsets, and getting rid of your limiting beliefs from the past. Step-by-step, you will achieve a very healthy brain and a powerful mind. If you are suffering from an unhealthy brain for any reason, then you may struggle to create a healthy mindset. This may be very difficult to deal with, but not impossible. It could even be possible that by creating a healthy, positive mindset, you may alleviate your suffering brain; remember, they are interconnected and work together.

And what about your paradigm, patterns, and habits?

Your mindset sets up your paradigm; it controls how you think about everything. A negative mindset creates a negative existence. It can sound scary, but you have the power to change this. That is exactly what the power of your mind is for! As an interconnected entity, by simply changing your thoughts, you will change your entire life, including your love life. Many couples give up when they are trying to rewire their way of thinking about sex. It is not about changing your partner's beliefs but assuming full responsibility towards updating the convictions that no longer work for you. We can see this fact in Eli and Chris case. Eli's paradigm saw sex as disgusting and as a wifely duty; as boring as doing laundry. Before she could improve her sex life, she had to work hard on changing her paradigm and beliefs about her sexuality first. Chris had to improve and update his beliefs as well.

Your paradigm controls your thoughts; your thoughts guide your brain; your brain controls your body chemistry and your behavior—and your actions determine your results. When changing your paradigm about love and sex, your goal is to be more and more convinced every day that it is healthy for you, for your partner, and for your relationship. This is the ultimate goal of sexual happiness and lovemaking. Once you re-set your mind and re-evaluate your beliefs about love, sex, and relationships, you will achieve a better mindset, leading to positive attitudes and realistic expectations. This trained mind-brain combo will help you to reach your relational goals to enjoy a positive love life in order to *make love 365 times a year*! Once you are aware of the interconnection of this amazing team—your mind and your brain—you will be ready to re-set them and open yourself up to all possibilities.

Part III: Building Mindsets

How do we know what makes up our mindsets about anything? How do we know what programs run our mindsets?

Step One: Acknowledge your mindsets by being aware of your automatic thoughts: what am I thinking? Think about what you are thinking. Many people go through life on autopilot. You must shut this off and pay attention to your thoughts so that your thoughts will become more conscious for you. This is what psychiatrist Dr. Aaron Beck, founder of Cognitive Behavioral Therapy (CBT) found—that beliefs are the root of peoples' problems. His techniques consist of teaching people to pay attention to what they say and believe to create change in their life.

This is especially true when you are dealing with everyday situations, particularly the ones that bother you. For example, if you are trying to change your mindset about food, you must be aware of your thoughts before, during, and after eating. If you are trying to change your mindset about sex, then you must be aware of your thoughts before, during, and after any sexual activity and intimate moments. In the case of Eli and Chris, the thoughts come when approaching sexual activities, so this is what needed to be changed.

Be aware of your daily thoughts about everything, especially your relationship. Ask yourself: what am I thinking? Is the situation making me confused or uncomfortable? Why? Think your thoughts! Be reasonable and logical. Think and think again! Your feelings are dictated by your thoughts; that is, you feel according to what you think. You feel your thoughts; you think and then feel.

Dr. Albert Ellis, PhD, founder of the Rational Emotive Behavioral Theory (REBT), explains in *Albert Ellis: Overcoming Destructive, Beliefs, Feelings, and Behaviors*, that "when people strongly desire to function productively and happily, and when Adversities (A) interfere with their doing so, they have Beliefs (B) about their desires and about their Adversities that result in emotional and behavioral Consequences (C) that are either largely unhealthy and self-defeating or largely healthy and self-helping."

This means that, we all react to adversities (A), but these reactions are different—they can be positive and healthy or negative and unhealthy—according to your belief system (B). Irrational Bs, which lead to self-defeating consequences, and Rational Bs, which lead to self-helping consequences, guide our emotions and actions. So, pay attention and remember the importance of your beliefs: they can help you and make you happy, or they can destroy you and make you very unhappy.

When Chris moved closer to Eli, she automatically thought he only wanted sex, when in fact he only wanted to connect to her. Becoming aware of these irrational thoughts is the first step to changing them. Keep track of your thoughts by recording observations in a journal or notebook. This technique will help you recognize the truth about your current unconscious mindset (your unconscious programs). When automatic thoughts are negative, they are called ANTs—Automatic Negative Thoughts—which I call "mental infections."

One big problem in the bedroom, causing all kinds of sexual issues, is the emergence of ANTs! They can get in the middle of your love life—and in your head—creating a disaster in the middle of your legs...

Step Two: Confrontation. After awareness, you can now confront your ANT's. Challenge your old beliefs and be totally honest to yourself. You can formulate questions that challenge the old beliefs, such as:

- ▶ Are my beliefs rational or irrational?
- ▶ Do I really like the way I think?
- ▶ Is this logical or illogical? Is this helping me?
- ▶ What are my expectations? Are they realistic?
- ▶ Can I have a different way of thinking?
- ▶ Are my views on sex and relationships influenced by my parents, my community, my religion, or my culture? Do I like them?
- ▶ What does this mean to me?
- ▶ Do I really want to change? What do I have to do differently? How scared am I?

You must become your own judge and take a serious evaluation of your actual paradigm, in a critical, constructive, honest, and responsible way. Do not lie to yourself! That will do nothing but hurt you in the long run.

After evaluating your mindset, if you realize that it is not what you want it to be (because it is nonsense, it is not helping you at all, or it is mostly negative) then continue with Step Three: reset your mindset!

Through conscious reprogramming, you can fill your mind with new, updated information that includes better experiences in your present, the reframing of negative past experiences, and the obtaining of objective-scientific evidence. This must be done as often as possible. I recommend doing it daily. You must find new facts and innovative ways of thinking and doing things. Update your information by continuing research, reading, and learning that can answer your questions and concerns. Don't settle with your old, negative, traditional, conventional or irrational beliefs and ideas. When you open yourself up to new, positive information, you open yourself up to a new mindset and to the possibility of *making love 365 times a year.*

Step Three: Reset your old mindset and create a new one. It is possible!

Remember Dr. Dweck, she advises: "You can change your mindset; it's about stretching yourself to learn something new. Developing yourself. Change isn't like surgery. The new beliefs take their place along-side the old ones, and as they become stronger, they give you a different way to think, feel, and act." Now see my ACR Steps: The Mindset Reset.

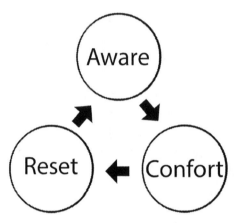

ACR Steps: The Mindset Reset

Resetting Your Mindset

There are many ways to re-set a mindset. I use three tools to re-set the mind: 1. The ability to focus. 2. The use of willpower 3. The creation of new, positive habits.

1. The Ability to Focus: What is focus? Focus is the ability to pay attention, to concentrate in on a single aspect of a task. It is a determination to do something. It is about keeping your eye on the target as you strive to meet the goal you set for yourself. Distraction is the opposite of focus. Beecham describes focus as "a visual concept, in the present tense—it's a 'now' concept. Where your eyes are focused is critical to your performance."

    We live in a time where it is easy to get distracted. The media, the news, the Internet, the virus, TV and smart phones at our fingertips most of the time. It's too much! It's easier to be distracted than to pay attention to the people and things that truly matter to us—our partner should be on the top of the list. If you are paying attention to outside distractions, it will be hard to focus. It's too much information for your brain to process—attempting to focus on one thing while also taking in the distractions around you.

In one of her great talks at the University of Santa Monica, Ariana Huffington, CEO of Thrive Global, said, "we are all, somehow, under the illusion that multitasking makes us more efficient. In fact, multitasking does not exist. It's really task-switching, and it's one of the most inefficient and stressful things we can do, and it also means that we miss life." Train yourself to focus on one task at a time, especially when you are in bed with your partner, so you can be more present and truly make love.

It is easy to get distracted by meaningless information, activities, and thoughts, not to mention your actual life responsibilities such as work, kids, housework, and all kinds of other duties. Your time with your partner should be precious. Focus on your partner when you are together as a couple and nothing else!

Attention! Paying attention to your partner is the key to connection! Everything you will read in this book directs you towards connection with your partner. The one way to master this connection is through your ability to focus. If you are paying attention to your partner daily, you can stay connected regardless of your adversities.

Use your attention to focus on your intentions. Intentions are crucial, but you must be clear and honest with yourself on what your deepest intentions are. What do you want out of your relationship?

Attention and intentions! Your attention is outside yourself—remember it like this: — "at"—tention is what you are focusing "at." On the other hand, in-tention is inside you, "in" yourself. I then see 'tention' like tension—a mental or emotional strain, an intense excitement. So, attention: intense excitement to outside of you; and intention: intense excitement to inside of you.

Your intention (in-side) is what should lead your attention (out-side), and, working together, attention and intention led to the fulfillment of your sex life and relationship goals. How can someone pay attention to something without an intention? They can't—it's a waste of energy! You will get everything except what really matters to you.

Likewise, an intention may vanish without the action of attention, another way of wasting energy! Attention and action are important to make your intention become a real possibility. Without attention, the intention may vanish through time. And, attention without intention is like a lost boat in the middle of the ocean. If you can't pay attention to or focus on your partner, it will be very hard to stay connected. You may live together but end up becoming platonic roommates.

Focus is a powerful force. To connect and stay connected to your beloved, you must focus on him or her. And make sure he or she also understands the importance of paying attention. You cannot make a connection with only one person focusing on the other. To create a strong connection through focus, you must be willing to GIVE attention with intention, RECEIVE attention with the same intention, and SHARE feelings, intentions, and attention with your beloved. Focusing on one another will then be the foundation of your connection and the cornerstone for staying in love—and *in lust*—over time.

I have found that three basic tasks are involved in achieving and mastering focus. These tasks are: A. know your target. B. Find meaning, and C. Concentrate.

A. Know your Target!

Your target is the "WHAT" of your equation. What is it that you want? Are you focusing on that? Have a sharp vision of what it is that you want. Don't worry about how and when it will happen, and just be clear on what it is that you want! Are you focusing on your past or on your present? Your present is your future. Have a vision.

B. Find Meaning!

Why do you want what you want? Are you focusing on that? If you have a reason, your focus has a purpose, and concentration will be much easier. Your whole experience must be meaningful and full of purpose. By understanding your situation, you can have a broad incentive for your continuing focus. Have meaning in your life.

C. Concentrate!

Concentration is the action of centering something. For example, centering your partner in your life means giving your relationship priority over other things. It is about giving direct attention, interest, and actions toward him or her so that your partner becomes your major concern or focus. At least your favorite!

A tip: make the whole process fun! The worst thing you can do is over complicate things. Relax and enjoy the journey while concentrating on your objective. Only through enjoyment will you be able to maintain your focus pleasantly. It is a strength you must develop to follow your intention to *make love 365 times a year.*

2. The Use of Willpower: Willpower is the ability to manage yourself through conscious determination and self-control. You must know how to calm and control yourself to achieve anything in life in a positive way, including your sexual happiness. Arnold Bennett wrote in *How to Live on Twenty-Four Hours a Day* that "mind control is the first element of a full existence."

Beecham is very knowledgeable about the conscious mind and its willpower. He says that "free will, drive, determination, and motivation are all by-products of the conscious mind...the conscious mind has the capacity to override the unconscious mind. The key keyword here is capacity. Sadly, most of us do not take advantage of this ability and instead function on autopilot."

Disciplining your mind with focus and attention will allow you to think about what is good for you while also recognizing your weaknesses. Charles Duhigg, author of *The Power of Habit*, wrote that "willpower isn't just a skill. It's a muscle, like the muscles in your arms or legs, and it gets tired as it works harder, so there's less power left for other things." Wang suggests that "willpower training involves some kind of activity to focus on, some mediating object that helps people stay focused and maintain attention." Everything is interconnected— focus, attention, willpower, discipline, and determination. We need all of that to sustain a vivid, healthy, and passionate love life and to *make love 365 times a year*!

Contrary to some beliefs, willpower is not about controlling others or being mean to people. In fact, it's impossible to control others or change them. Manipulation, punishment, intimidation, threats, pressure, and coercion are harmful attempts to control others. Instead, use positive persuasion, encouragement, inspiration, reassurance, and seduction because these are positive ways to induce changes, influence others, and attract attention. It is never about controlling anyone. In Chapter 6, we will discuss the power of seduction as an important tool to provoke and attract your partner sexually. Again, it is never about controlling your partner, but nicely persuading them.

If you try to change your partner, you will only meet defeat. Every person should be responsible for and able to change or improve themselves. Changes, modifications, or improvements are very personal and unique to each individual person. You may suggest, recommend, or influence your partner or others, and they may choose to follow up on your suggestions or not. It is totally up to them. If you work on yourself first and modify your mindset through focus and willpower, your partner will most likely observe what you're doing and will make an effort to improve him or herself as well.

A recent study asked 5,000 people to change one of their behaviors. In the end, only 600 people could successfully change. That's only 12% of participants could change. Why? According to the researchers, out of 5,000 people, only 600 understood the power of self-control (willpower) and used it! That's proof that you really can change your beliefs and behaviors, but it isn't easy. Willpower is absolutely needed for any change to occur. This study concluded that most people had a low capacity to control their behavior. They attempted to change outside factors instead of looking inward.

The real power is in acknowledging your weaknesses, controlling and improving them. But, if you put your effort toward other people, such as your partner, you may eventually feel like they are controlling you. You are misusing your power and missing the whole point if you focus on others instead of on yourself.

Your parents, your partner, your children, society, religion, and people who surround you have the potential to try to control you if you are unaware that the real power is within you and only in you! Sometimes, we desire to tell others what to do—which is easy—but having them instead tell us what to do, may cause conflict. In fact, it is much harder to control yourself than it is to try to control others around you. Only through your willpower can you make lasting changes.

Think about this: If your partner is angry, why do you have to be angry too? Does having a distraught boss mean you also have to be distraught? Owning your feelings and thoughts without pretending to change others' feelings is also a way to have self-control.

Resistance is the only thing that stands between you and what you want to change. When progressing to the next level, you may meet resistance. Be aware that your internal resistance will take the form of excuses, such as: "I'm tired," "it's too hard," "I don't like it," "I can't," "tomorrow," "you make me this way," "they are standing on my way," and so on. These excuses are focused on outside factors—distractions—and stand between you and your happiness. Control yourself regardless of everyone else. Only then can you change yourself and your circumstances so that things will improve.

3. The Creation of New, Positive Habits: What are habits? Habits are patterns, behaviors, and ways to do things that you create, usually unconsciously, that in turn create you. You are your habits! This is a never-ending cycle, from acts learned unconsciously that might be unhealthy, to conscious acts that are healthy for you, which will become unconscious again as you get used to them.

Duhigg explains that "the routine occurs by habit…habits, scientists say, emerge because the brain is constantly looking for ways to save effort. Left to its own devices, the brain will try to make almost any routine into a habit, because habits allow our minds to ramp down more often. This effort-saving instinct is a huge advantage."

As I mentioned, this is a never-ending cycle that goes from unconscious to conscious, to unconscious again. All of this is great if your habits are positive and work for you as a positive invisible force. Now, what if they aren't so great? It is a problem if you are unaware of a negative invisible force that makes you behave against your own best interests. The problem does not have to be too bad if you practice awareness and pay attention to your daily habits in order to consciously change them for better ones, until they become unconscious and work for you. The work ahead is to consciously create new healthy habits—in this case, love habits—to create a new sexual you, the greatest you possible: successful, loving, and sexually happy!

Now, how do we create new love habits? It looks simple, but it is not. Remember, the first step is to realize how these habits were created in order to create new ones. You first created your old habits when you were very young—your family and the culture surrounding you. This was done without your awareness; you did it without knowing you were forming habits. You followed them without realizing it, like a robot would follow commands.

Most people believe and say, "I'm that way": lazy, explosive, angry, non-affectionate, non-sexual, low drive, emotionally unavailable, unfaithful, and so on. It's fatalistic thinking to believe you can't change the way you are and how you do things. In fact, it's your habits that made you behave the way you do. You are not "that way;" you behave according to your habits. If you change your habits, you can change the way you do things and transform yourself for the better. It is not about changing "YOU"; it's about making a "BETTER YOU." You can no longer be "that way" anymore. You will be YOUR BEST SELF.

Those old habits molded the person you are today. We all have done this unconsciously, until the need for changes and improvements came and forced us to establish new and better habits in a conscious way. Yes, habits are that powerful, so use it to your favor and get rid of the habits that are working against your love life.

Ask yourself now the following questions:

▶ What are my goals?
▶ Is my goal to have a fulfilling sex life?
▶ Is it to be sexually happy?

Let's create new love habits to behave accordingly by improving your new sexual mindset. How can you act differently if you haven't changed your mindset? Remember, it's a cycle. You create your habits, and these habits, in turn, create you. So, set up new habits by doing things differently than usual. Remember your intentions, so your new love habits will help you towards your goal. At first, it will be hard work because you are accustomed to doing things a certain way. It takes courage and requires intense focus, willpower, self-control, determination, and discipline.

But once you accomplish your goal—the formation of a new love habit—it will be easy and relaxing, as Gretchen Rubin, bestselling author, describes in *Better than Before*: "habits make change possible by freeing us from decision making and using self-control." It is as simple as letting it flow naturally, consciously. In this way, you may experience your new habits even without realizing it. So, make sure you choose your new habits well, especially your new love habits, through use of your new positive mindset, so that you will naturally *make love 365 times a year.*

Duhigg suggests a formula to change habits: 1: Identify your routine and change it. 2: Use rewards. 3: Identify the cue. And 4: Have a plan. As Duhigg explains, "a habit is a formula our brain automatically follows: When I see CUE, I will do ROUTINE to get a REWARD. To re-engineer that formula, we need to begin making choices again."

Author of *The 5 Second Rule*, Mel Robbins, has proposed a fascinating method to stop your ANTs (Automatic Negative Thoughts) and overcome your old negative habits. According to Robbins, you can "think about things that bring you joy instead of focusing on the negative. Start by counting backwards to yourself: 5-4-3-2-1. The counting will help you focus on the goal or commitment and distract you from the worries, thoughts, and fears in your mind. The Rule will quiet your self-doubt and build confidence as you push yourself to pursue your passions." This is true, especially if you haven't established a new strong mindset yet.

Use *The 5 Second Rule* whenever you need to push yourself. Your new habits will change your life. Changing the habits that aren't working for you is a big step towards a more satisfying relationship and a happier sex life. If you feel insecure, unloved, misunderstood, or unsatisfied in your relationship, it is probably because you are not aware of the actions and habits you have formed, leading to distress and disconnection.

Remember, your beliefs—rational or irrational—will lead to either satisfaction and happiness or dissatisfaction and unhappiness in times of adversity and conflict. This applies to all aspects of life, including sex and relationships, and applies to both members of the relationship. Yes, you can establish better habits, regulate yourself, and change for good, but what about your partner? They are part of the relationship, too, and will affect you if you don't work together as a team. Remember Eli and Chris? They both suffered as well.

Throughout life, you will face contradictions and problems within your relationship—it is normal. Your new love habits will help you successfully overcome them while maintaining the connection. Your new habits will become your new behavior, which is the manifestation of your new mindset, thoughts, and feelings. This cycle takes time, but it is the way to make permanent changes. Only by changing limiting and maladaptive habits will your relationship and sex life improve. This amazing, never-ending cycle of working on these three skills (the ability to focus, the use of willpower, and the creation of new love habits) will bring you the connection you deserve in order to *make love 365 times a year*. It's worth doing!

And once you have done it—VOILA! When life changes, you will have better love habits to deal with different situations in your relationship. By creating your new positive mindset, you have created a way to enjoy your love life regardless of external circumstances around you.

Part IV: Your Sexual Mindset

What do you *think* about sex and sexuality? Are you confusing intimacy with sex? Are you aware of your thoughts and beliefs about sex? Can you describe your sex-related belief system? Is it like that of your parents or childhood caregivers? How has your religion, community, and peers affected your beliefs about relationship and sexuality?

What does intimacy *mean* to you? Sexuality? Sex? Passion? Romance? Love? Being in a relationship? Being monogamous? What do you think about frequent sexual activity? About orgasms? What do you think about *making love 365 times a year*? Do you think it is possible? What does your partner think? Do you feel connected to your partner? What does connection mean to you?

A healthy *sexual* mindset is the foundation of any satisfactory, healthy sex life. It is my first secret, Sex Secret #1. Without a positive sexual mindset, it won't be possible to surrender to the arms of Eros, the Greek God of Love, and *make love 365 times a year*. Without a belief system about the greatness of sexuality, positive sexual thoughts, and positive sexual attitudes, a person can hardly sexually function, let alone fully enjoy and have pleasure during intimate sexual experiences. And not to mention their ability to frequently make love.

To craft your sexual mind, start by asking yourself some questions about sex—and please don't lie to yourself:

- ▶ Am I aware of my sexual thoughts?
- ▶ Do I have them?
- ▶ Do I have sexual fantasies? Do I allow and enjoy them?
- ▶ What prevents me from thinking about sex?
- ▶ Am I in control of my sexual thoughts, or do they control me?
- ▶ What do I think about having sex? About making love, about making love with my partner. Do I feel comfortable around them?
- ▶ Do I have the desire to have sex? With whom? When?
- ▶ Have I ever thought about not having sex? How does that make me feel?
- ▶ Do I masturbate? What are my beliefs about it? Do I feel comfortable masturbating? Why not? What turns me on? What turns me off?
- ▶ Do I know what my partner thinks about all these questions?

It is okay if you have answered negatively to some of these questions. The idea is that you will become aware of your core beliefs about sexuality, confront them, and change them to improve your love life. So, keep this in mind: you may be okay with a poor sex life or with not having sex at all, but what about your partner? When growing your sexual mindset, think about them and your relationship as well—you are not alone! As Dweck says, "in relationships, two more things enter the picture—your partner and the relationship itself." You, your partner, and your relationship can grow and change for good. And those changes begin in your mind.

In 2017, the 23rd Congress for the World Association of Sexual Health (WAS) was held in Prague. I was very honored to be able to attend and participate. During the congress, some of the lectures highly emphasized the importance of establishing a sexual mind for the optimization of sexual desire, especially among women.

One of the participants lecturing about fantasies and sexual desire was Dr. Maria Sophocles, a board-certified Ob/Gyn. Dr. Sophocles explained that "for women, the beginning is their own unblocking of the mind and being open to sexual thoughts," in order to have sexual desire and enjoy their sexuality. Dr. Jaqueline Brendler, a renowned Brazilian gynecologist and sexologist, was also an important speaker on sexual desire and the mind. I share Brendler's findings: "for people with low libido, desire is not activated by touching; we cannot use tact to activate desire, it's first activated by thoughts. I use the "Think About Sex" task in women with low libido. Sexual desire is activated through touch and works very well only in healthy women."

Brendler then developed a technique called *Menu for Sex*, a repertoire of erotic scenes, which was first published in SRBSH 2005 (a Scientific Society of Studies in Human Sexuality). These techniques are based on helping women to think about sex daily. So, "women will have their time to restore sexual desire before any sexual behavior. Desire, when motivated by "thinking about sex," even though it is less commonly known among women, can be easily learned, far away from the pressures of the sexual act itself," emphasized Brendler.

Both speakers agreed—when a woman with low libido doesn't desire sex, she should no longer be touched sexually, avoiding the pressure to engage in sexual activities. This will only worsen their situation. Women with sexual desire issues must, first and foremost, work on their thoughts. Be aware that touch is not recommended, whereas the development of a sexual mindset is, when restoring sexual desire via the think about sex method. That means that by creating a sexual mindset first, individuals with low libido can reactivate the desire for sex in order to enjoy it more. Therefore, Sex Secret #1 is all about having a healthy sexual mindset.

In fact, without a healthy sexual mindset—a belief system that allows us to be sexual in the appropriate context—we aren't free to spontaneously engage in pleasurable sexual activities of any kind. If you are doing the opposite, you'll probably reject sex or only engage in it to please your partner, as Eli did. So, you will end up detaching from yourself, from your genitals, and from your sexual feelings, just to "get through sex"—the old "lay back and think of England" trick. Once again, without a healthy sexual mindset, no one can fully enjoy sex for pleasure and connection, and to *make love 365 times a year...*

Now, what about passion?! When you have established a healthy sexual mindset, your desire for sex increases—desire comes from your mind, not from your genitals—as well as your energy to pursue more sex. That, to me, is where passion comes from—from desire and wanting more of something good—enjoying and wanting more pleasurable sex.

Passion is all about wanting, and wanting is desire, and desire is curiosity. If you cannot imagine something, how can you want it? For example, if you want food, such as a slice of cake, you imagine it first, if you don't have it near you; then you begin to want it, and only then do you eat the cake. Without that first thought that creates the desire, you never go after the cake. It's the same for lovemaking...

Usually, among men, I have found the opposite; sometimes they think TOO MUCH about their sexual performance to the point of creating all kinds of sexual problems, such as Anticipatory Anxiety. For example, as explained by psychologist and sexologist Jack Morin, PhD, "preoccupation with performance can cause people to shift their attention permanently from the pleasures of sex to the potentials of failure."

With our case couple, Eli and Chris, we saw that Eli wouldn't even think about sex. She did not have a sexual mind yet. Because she would not even think about it, she could not feel the desire that leads to action—neither the action that leads to wanting more. Once a woman reestablishes her desires for sex, the touching will follow, and thus the passion. If you want a satisfactory sex life full of passion, then you need to establish a positive sexual mindset. Remember, your beliefs, ideas, and feelings make your reality. Reality is all subjective. By modifying your belief system and your paradigm, you modify your reality.

What about your expectations? Can expectations be modified as well? Yes! Your expectations depend on your beliefs, and this is very important for your sexual happiness. Your sexual happiness is the byproduct of your expectations and your perception.

Sexual Expectations

Sexual expectations are based on three factors:

1. Your environment: What your environment has taught you about sex. Your parents, family, friends, and all the people around you may influence your attitudes towards sex. This includes the impact of religion, media, your cultural/social network, the Internet (including porn), education, and everything around you that may have helped you create a set of beliefs about sex.

2. Your past experiences: From non-experience, to all your experiences that have involved sexual feelings and/or sexual activities—that is, everything you have learned from being with other people (whether of the same or opposite sex). This also includes your feelings of love, lust, hate, disgust, happiness, pleasure, and so on. Negative sexual experiences or sexual traumas may have a very negative impact on your sexual expectations. Your past experiences or inexperience, positive or negative, has helped to create your beliefs system.

3. Your self-knowledge: The experience you have with your own self when masturbating or being sexual in any way (including sexual fantasies, thoughts, dreams, desires, and behavior). The knowledge of experiencing your own sexuality impacts your belief system as well.

Your expectations based on these three factors can be poor, unrealistic, negative, and unhealthy; or they can be positive, rich, healthy, and realistic. They can be high, moderate, or low as well. When your expectations (thoughts) match your perception (what you are living), then you feel satisfied. But, when your expectations (what you believe) do not match your perception, you will feel unsatisfied, even with the best lover on earth!

Therefore, to be sexually satisfied and fully enjoy your sex life, or any sexual activity, you must be very careful with your expectations! False, wrong, and unrealistic expectations based on your past experiences can be detrimental to your love life.

My suggestion is this: Don't have expectations at all, or at least lower them, while making love. Just be present in the moment to experience and *feel* every time you are with your partner or with yourself. Expect to have no expectations and enjoy the moment! Your perception will always match your expectations. Satisfaction guaranteed!

Work on building a powerful sexual mindset that allows you to be sexually free without restrictions, so you can enjoy your thoughts and fantasies, and engage in consensual, healthy, responsible, and pleasurable sexual activities, with no expectations. That is not to say you must think about sex 24/7, but you must have the ability to think about sex whenever you need it. You should be able to turn yourself on, to know your likes and dislikes, and to have your own sexual fantasies repertoire.

Without a healthy sexual mindset, you may not sustain passion. Once you have set your sexual mind up to think freely about sex, your brain will release the right chemicals and hormones that you need to be ready to make love. Remember, the mind & brain are interconnected. Your brain will automatically do what it needs to do, according to the mind's messages. Be sure you are aware of your mind messages! Don't let it go on autopilot if your sexual mind isn't ready.

Sexologist and past president of the World Association for Sexual Health (WAS), Dr. Eusebio Rubio-Aurioles, MD, PhD, points out in most of his speeches around the world the importance of knowledge in our sex lives. He emphasizes that "facts free your love life." Healthy sexual minds are built through knowledge, and sexual knowledge is a sexual right that should be available to all. Sexual information and facts are valuable to anyone eager to improve, modify, reconstruct, or re-build a sexual mindset. Without appropriate knowledge, fears and doubts about sex will take over the mind. We fear what we don't know.

Eli, because of the poor sexual mindset she adopted from her parents, was pushing away, rejecting, and avoiding her husband's sexual approaches. She was thinking about romantic, idealistic love, denying any sexual feelings and labeling them as wrong and evil. Healthy sexuality cannot be reached without a healthy sexual mindset based on facts, knowledge, and positive experiences. We first adopt our parents' beliefs about sex. Now, we must build our own paradigm about sex. No therapy or program can work if you have a sexually closed mind. But anything can be accomplished if your mind is open and ready to instruct your brain. It is the foundation for a healthy sex life. Reset, and the rest will follow!

This is the reason why my Sex Secret #1 is the MIND! Let's work on building an amazing, healthy, and beautiful sexual mindset, the one you need for a fulfilling love life and to *make love 365 times a year.* I want you to realize that there are a lot of facts available to you, through the media, books, and therapists.

You don't have to wait for a certain time or watch porn to accomplish this (porn is ONLY for adult entertainment, not for education). Just open your mind and relax!

Creating a Healthy Sexual Mindset

You, first, need to understand that you—and all humans—are sexual beings, from birth to death. You are a sexual being! Never forget this! From birth until death, there is not a day that goes by that you are not a sexual being. Be grateful every day that you are a sexual being. Think about how happy you are—EVERY DAY—to have a sexual relationship with yourself and with your partner.

Second, you must have the belief that you can be sexually active at any time in your life. It's okay; you're not broken. Your genitals are a part of you. They aren't gross or wrong as well as your fluids. They are fun, great, and normal!

Then, choose positive thoughts about sex. Think about sex three or four times a day. Pick a time or a place to think about any pleasant sexual image you can recall something enjoyable from an erotic movie, past hot experiences, or a fantasy. You can choose to think about it in the shower, right before bed, or on Saturday mornings, but take your time to think about your sexuality in a healthy, positive, and constructive way. Be grateful for it!

Masturbation, or solo sex, plays a significant role in the creation of a healthy sexual mindset. It is the foundation of your sexuality. Your sexuality is who you are. Through solo sex, you can discover your own way to sexual satisfaction.

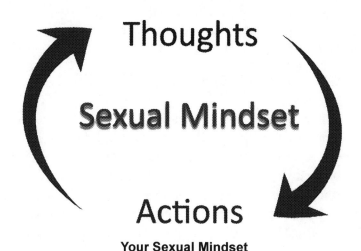

Your Sexual Mindset

Sex is as important as love is for your relationship! A healthy relationship needs sex, love, intimacy, and lust to be combined in a harmonically balanced and intertwined way—we will talk about this in Chapter 3. There is nothing better than a satisfying love life. As Dweck mentioned, "a good, lasting relationship comes from effort and from working through inevitable differences," and many times these are sexual differences. But by growing and modifying your sexual mindsets together, these differences can be lessened.

Lovemaking is love in action—doing love—as I say! It is the physical manifestation of the love you feel for each other. Through your whole body, you can express that love to show how much you care and how much you want each other. It is the deepest connection a couple can experience. It is about love and freedom. "Connectivity drives love," as one of my clients told me in a session.

To create sexual gratitude, have a set of positive affirmations to tell yourself every morning. Affirmations are an important step toward the creation of any mindset, including a sexual mindset. For instance, sex coach Pia Battaglia, author of *The Book of Sexontological Affirmations*, suggests affirmations to help you create a positive sexual mindset. Here are a few of her affirmations as well as other positive thoughts to choose from. Feel free to add more—anything that works for you:

> "I am a healthy sexual being."
> "I am thankful for being a sexual being."
> "I am thankful for my partner, spouse, or the one to come."
> "I appreciate and love my genitals."
> "I appreciate and love my partner's genitals."
> "My sexuality is precious, priceless, and I respect that."
> "Sex is good, healthy, and brings me joy."
> "I am sexually attractive."
> "My sexual happiness is important to me."

Start with affirmations you are comfortable with, then build up to ones you are less comfortable with. Begin to believe that this is your new reality, a real thing; your conscious and unconscious mind will start believing it. You have that ability. Just do it! Using the tools listed in the mindset section and my recommendations, you can start creating your sexual mindset right away! Positively thinking about sex—with no shame, guilt, or fear—will change your paradigm. Then you will follow it, creating new habits that will make things much easier for you. Being sexually active will keep you deeply connected to your partner. Think about the meaning of that!

For me, *making love 365 times a year,* and being sexually happy are the best ways to stay healthy, keep my immune system strong, and be connected to my partner—Pedro. It is beyond imagination! I know it is possible, and I know that any couple can do the same, but it requires some work and effort. The 7 *Sex Secrets* are here to help you so that lovemaking will always be possible.

I also walked the path and worked intensely to create my sexual mindset long ago. Then, I made sure that Pedro and I shared the same beliefs about love, sex, and relationships—at least 80% of them. Otherwise, this amazing sex life that we enjoy every day wouldn't be possible.

While you are thinking about your new positive sexual thoughts, be aware of how they make you feel. When saying your affirmations or spending time thinking about sex, what are your reactions? Do you feel anger, sadness, happiness, shame, joy, guilt, or freedom? If you are having negative reactions, try to understand why, and where these reactions come from.

You should only feel good! So, relax and associate these sexual thoughts with pleasurable sensations such as pleasant smells or fun memories. If this is too difficult for you, find professional help, but don't leave it unaddressed. Addressing fears, anxieties, and worries is part of the process. The idea is to only associate sexuality with positive experiences, pleasure, and fun. Avoid pushing or making yourself feel obligated while building your new sexual paradigm; a healthy sexual mind is NOT a punishment; it is a blessing.

Then, you can feel confident! Once you are confident, allow yourself to go beyond your mental comfort zone. Let yourself imagine sexual scenarios that may arouse you and bring you pleasure. There is nothing to fear within your mind. This is what freedom truly is. As you imagine more and more, your comfort zone will expand and change. Your comfort zone is elastic; you can expand it to become more comfortable with different topics and scenarios. This will allow you to explore sexual thoughts while feeling secure and safe. After you become comfortable with your sexual thoughts, it will be time for some responsible and loving action!

Once you begin to feel good and move beyond your comfort zone, it's time to decide how far you want to go. What are your limits? Know these and find them without fear. Then you can feel secure about yourself in a sexual way. Decide what your goals are. What do you want to explore? In that way, you will create a respectful sexual mindset, the one you appreciate, recognize, and pursue. Explore by yourself first. Remember, masturbation or solo sex will help you know what feels good and help you decide what you are comfortable with. Don't limit yourself!

Morin explains in *The Erotic Mind* the reasons why many people have a very restricted paradigm and feel so bad and guilty about sex. He says that "many people grew up in homes so permeated with anti-sexual restrictions that the drama of violating prohibitions has become the central feature of their eroticism. These people are prisoners of sexual prohibition…"

Yes, prisoners of an obsolete, unhealthy mindset! Now, as an adult, "you have grown sufficiently free to use prohibitions for your own enjoyment and play," advises Morin. That is, you now have the capacity to build a new, conscious, and positive sexual mindset that sets you up freely for a healthy sexuality.

Knowing how to use your sexual mind to turn on your body is your responsibility now. If you don't know how to have an orgasm by yourself, how can you expect your partner to know how to please you? Have orgasms without guilt! Learn to enjoy it, relax, and free yourself. You now possess a healthy sexual mindset to support you; what else do you need? When you feel good about your sexual mindset, your own body, and enjoy solo sex, you can implement what you have learned with your partner. Explore all the possibilities that may work for you and enjoy together your new sexual mindsets!

The most important thing is to be calm, comfortable, and to have fun! Psychologist and sex therapist in Los Angeles, Dr. Shannon Chavez says that "sex is a serious part of overall health and well-being, but it doesn't have to be serious to the point of lacking play and fun. If you're not having fun, it can turn serious and lead to you criticizing yourself or your partner."

Beecham also advises, "once the belief changes from 'I can't do this very well' to 'I think I can do this if I change,' then the actual behaviors and outcomes change. The beliefs that you have about yourself and your abilities are not facts. They are your tightly held opinions." So, be strong enough to endure sexual changes and transformation. I believe that consistency, commitment, and discipline bring success. You have now the MOST essential element: Sex Secret #1: A heathy sexual mindset," to fully love and *make love 365 times a year!*

"If you can imagine it, you can achieve it. If you
can dream it, you can become it."
—William Arthur Ward.

Part V: Seven Simple Suggestions & Recommended Sources

7 Simple Suggestions for a Sexual Mindset

1. Deeply meditate by yourself (reflect): What are the precise messages you are sending to your brain regarding sex, sexuality, relationships, and love in general? How strong, or foggy, is your message?

2. Ask yourself the following questions and then ask your partner:

   ▶ Is my mindset helping me? Do I have a sexual mindset? What is my partner's mindset?
   ▶ What are my sexual goals?
   ▶ Why do I think this way?
   ▶ Are my views on sex and relationships the same as those of my parents, my community, my religion?
   ▶ What does this mean to me? To my partner? Are we sexually happy?
   ▶ What does this mean to me?
   ▶ How have my past experiences impacted me?
   ▶ Is my goal to have a fulfilling sex life?
   ▶ To be sexually happy?
   ▶ Do I have sexual fantasies? Do I allow and enjoy them?
   ▶ What prevents me from thinking about sex?
   ▶ Am I in control of my sexual thoughts, or do they control me?
   ▶ What do I think about having sex? About making love? About making love with my partner?
   ▶ Do I have the desire to have sex?
   ▶ Have I ever thought about not having sex? How does that make me feel?
   ▶ Do I masturbate? What are my beliefs about it? Do I feel comfortable masturbating?
   ▶ Do I know how my partner thinks about all these questions?

3. Choose to consciously think about SEX 3 or 4 times a day. Choose times when you can fantasize and imagine, and think about sex, and

having sex every day, as normal as being as normal as having a good meal. Feel free to imagine whatever you'd like; it is only in your mind! Remember: "If you can imagine it, you can achieve it."

4. Create a repeat set of positive daily sexual affirmations. They are up to you, and for you. Preferably, repeat them as soon as you wake up or right before going to sleep in a comfortable, relaxing way. Be sure to be grateful for being sexual.

5. Always remember that sexual health and good sex come from your BRAIN. For instance, your interest in sex and your sexual energy are regulated by the dopamine in your brain. And your brain needs direction (information), among other things, to release the right chemicals.

6. Learn to think first, then make decisions, and then flow and feel. Remember Beecham: "The mind unconsciously is set to this tempo and will repeat it automatically. A big part of success training involves truly understanding why you are doing what you are doing, how to do it, and what it is you are doing." So, get instructed, re-think your thoughts, and learn new positive information about healthy sexuality.

7. When in bed with your partner, keep the focus on the moment, the here and now. Be present, be there, and intensify your focus with your willpower and intentions, and nothing else. Practice focus when making love.

Recommended Sources for Sex Secret #1

Albert Ellis: Overcoming Destructive, beliefs, Feelings, and Behaviors by Dr. Albert Ellis, Ph.D.

Resurrecting Sex by Dr. David Schnarch

Mindset: The New Psychology of Success by Carol S. Dweck, Ph.D.

The Power of Habit: Why We Do What We Do in Life and Business by Charles Duhigg

How to live on 24 hours a day by Arnold Bennett

The 5 Second Rule by Mel Robbins

Better than Before by Gretchen Rubin

Elite Minds by Dr. Stan Beecham

How People Change by Marion Solomon and Daniel J. Siegel

The Erotic Mind: Unlocking the Inner Sources of Sexual Passion and Fulfillment by Jack Morin, Ph.D.

The Neuroscience of Everyday Life—from *The Great Courses*—by Professor Dr. Sam Wang

Dr. Eusebio Rubio A. Asociacion Mexicana para la Salud Sexual, A.C. Website: www.amssac.org

Sexual Menu. Abstracts of the 17th World Congress of Sexology, and *Mapping What Increases Sexual Arousal in Heterosexual Women* by Dr. Jaqueline, Brendler (Portuguese)

The Book of Sexontological Affirmations by Pia Battaglia (Spanish & English)

SEX SECRET
2

CHAPTER 2

A Healthy Lifestyle

➤—╫————◦╈▷

Don't knock masturbation—it's sex with someone I love.
—Woody Allen

Part I: The Relationship with Yourself

A quote from Lucille Ball that I like says: "Love yourself first, and everything else falls into line. You really have to love yourself to get anything done in this world." I share that thought all the time; nothing can be done without self-love, which is sometimes confused with selfishness. Dr. Ava Cadell, PhD, leading love guru, author of eight books and founder of Loveology University, says in *Neuroloveology* that "no matter what challenges life may have given you, before anyone will be able to truly love you, you have to be able to comfortably and confidently say four things:

1. I am worthy of love.
2. I am worthy of happiness.
3. I am worthy of respect.
4. I am worthy of great sex—Yes, GREAT SEX."

Caring for your body is a physical manifestation of the love you have for yourself, because your body is a vital part of you. If you truly love yourself, you should treat your body well. Taking proper care of our bodies is a direct response to feeling worthy. Don't get me wrong—I don't want you to be worried about your body, per se, but about its health. Your body, as Emily Nagoski, PhD, Director of Wellness Education at Smith College and author of *Come as You Are*, "is normal...we all have the same parts but organized differently." Pay attention instead to the well-being of your unique and beautiful body!

A well-treated body (to the best extent possible) is key to a successful sex life and to *make love 365 times a year*! Remember, sex is something you do—a behavior—and you do it with your body; so, sex then is a bodily activity. Your goal here is to love, respect, accept, and appreciate your whole self, including your body with its genitals—the only one you have. So, let's make sure your body has life and energy, and that it is as healthy as possible, regardless of your age, gender, or physical limitations.

Let's learn now from a new case: Sarah and Frank, a couple with an unhealthy lifestyle that almost killed their sex life.

Case #2: Sarah & Frank

Sarah and Frank had no obvious problems in their relationship. They loved each other, had a good family, were okay financially, both had a positive sexual mindset (Sex Secret #1). They did not mind discussing sex with me at all and were very attracted to one another.

But they still weren't having "the sex we desired," according to them.

They had been married for nine years and dated for two years before that. Both worked; Sarah was 36, and Frank was 37. They had one child, a son, who was eight years old.

We immediately began talking about sex, and they explained they didn't have any negative attitudes, beliefs, or hang-ups about sex. They freely discussed touching one another, watching porn occasionally, and the good sex they'd had earlier in their relationship.

But that was before their son. And the mortgage. And bad habits. The demanding jobs and the many stresses of their life led them towards an unhealthy lifestyle. So, I began to ask more about their day to day life. To find the problem, I had them share their typical routines and difficulties outside the bedroom.

"I've got type I diabetes," Frank finally told me. When asked what he does to treat it, he just shrugged me off. "I still eat what I want. I walk a bit around for exercise and in my job, that's about it. I usually feel pretty tired."

When pressed, he admitted he wasn't controlling his diabetes or taking good care of himself at all. I turned to Sarah, and she agreed.

"We eat terribly. Him more than me, but I know I'm overweight," she said. She admitted she hated exercising and refused to do any kind of physical movement at all. Then, I asked her about her body-image.

"I'm fat I don't like much how I look," she said, shaking her head. "I don't like how I look," she insisted again. "And I've been having a lot of headaches and stomach aches lately. I just don't feel like doing anything; I have pretty low energy too, always feel tired, so...."

"That's why we can't have sex; she doesn't feel like it," Frank added.

"I can't help it; I feel like an old lady!" she answered.

I hear this a lot in my practice, and as an almost 55-year-old woman, hearing someone in their 30s say they're old is always a shock!

"I've had panic attacks too," Sarah told me.

I asked what brought on the panic attacks, and she pointed at Frank.

"He wants to have sex and be intimate, even when both feel tired," she complained. "When I say I can't, he gets frustrated. I can't help that I'm falling asleep all the time. Then when he gets mad, I start having panic attacks. I feel tired even to please myself... I know it's wrong, but that's the truth."

By now, I knew what was happening. Both Sarah and Frank seem shocked when I tell them that their unhealthy lifestyle is directly causing their unfulfilling sex life. They had never connected these unhealthy habits with their sex problems! But when your body is unhealthy, your sex life may be unhealthy as well.

You can have a fantastic sexual mindset, but if your mindset about lifestyle is bad, your body—and your sex life—will suffer.

As we were talking, I saw their unhealthy lifestyle unfold:

1. Bad eating habits

"We love McDonald's," Frank explained. "Really any fast food, but McDonald's hamburgers especially."

They also eat mostly bread, pasta, and sugar. Rarely is there any nutritious or healthy eating in their household. "No time for preparing healthy meals," both explained.

2. Refusal to exercise

Especially Sarah, who just kept saying how much she hated exercise. Both "feel too tired for working out."

3. Inadequate sleep

This was baffling to me at first, but Sarah explained their son didn't sleep well, so she felt unable to sleep as well. She worried about her son, which lead her to wake up a lot at night, or even to let their son sleep with them in the same bed!

4. Too much work without any fun—even no masturbation.

On the weekends they spent Saturday shopping with their son and Sunday going to church, which they both admitted to finding stressful. "It's a duty," Sarah said when I asked. "But we don't get anything out of it." They never spend fun time together; they did not create room in their lives for a better lifestyle, or for their own sex life!

Their sex life had suffered because of their bad eating habits, stress, fatigue, lack of exercise, and poor sleep. And now it was not enough for them. Different people, different couples, require different things out of their relationship. And both Frank and Sarah required more than they were currently getting.

Frank and Sarah's unhealthy lifestyles had led to a low self-image that kept them from having sex. Sarah hated having sex because of how she looked, and she and Frank both hated it because of fatigue.

"I want to have sex; I desire him, but I don't feel sexy enough," she said. "I don't want him to see my belly or my butt."

"I don't care about it!" Frank said.

"But I do," Sarah countered.

As their self-esteem and confidence lowered, their desire to have sex lowered as well as their sexual frequency. Once sex became "a problem," they started avoiding it.

Let's go back to thinking of your body as a car, a vehicle. Even if you have a positive sexual mindset, but your body (the vehicle) is not functioning as it should, you may have difficulty moving towards action and doing what you want to do. This does not mean that you cannot enjoy your sexual mind and have pleasure, it means that you will have to look for ways—there are plenty different ways—to help your body (the vehicle) to go and experience your desires.

Remember from Chapter 1, how important your mind is to your sex life. Think of it like this—your mind is your GPS, and your body is your vehicle. The GPS cannot go without a car, but without the GPS, the car might get lost. A healthy brain and a sexual mind (GPS) are needed to direct a body (the vehicle) for healthy sexual expressions (destiny).

In all aspects of life—your love life, your work life, your family life—you must take care of YOURSELF FIRST. You will find it impossible to take care of others if you are not in working order yourself! Think about the last time you were on an airplane. Flight attendants always tell you to place your oxygen mask on first before placing an oxygen mask on others traveling with you, be they your kids, parents, or partner. You cannot help another unless you are able to breathe first.

Be aware of yourself as an intellectual, spiritual, emotional, and sexual being. You are a complex, multi-faceted human. Consider ALL aspects of yourself and fulfill them. Not only one or two of them, but all. One essential aspect is the physical—your body. Your body needs nutrition, water, sleep, and rest to better function. By exercising, eating right, sleeping well, having fun, laughing, and having sex you will improve your overall health, boost your immune system, and lift up your self-esteem—you will feel better about yourself—to be able to fully enjoy your love life.

Do not neglect yourself, please! It is never too late! A great example of this is the experience of my father: At age 69 he was ill and giving up on his happiness. He then decided to take massive action to get healthier and stronger—he did it. Years later, he got remarried and was able to fully enjoy his new life, and sex life with his new partner, because of his improved bodily condition. I witnessed how through continued effort and willpower my father was able to improve his poor physical conditions to enjoy, as much as he could, his love life and make love again. He took care of himself first to feel better and live longer.

If you are not capable of loving yourself, how will you truly love your partner? How will your partner love you? If you do not have a good relationship with yourself, how can you have a good relationship with your partner? You must love yourself unconditionally to be available for your partner and experience a pleasurable love life. You can improve your self-esteem, your overall health, the way you talk to yourself, and your confidence. Knowing yourself sexually is part of loving yourself and is essential to fully enjoy your sex life. Anything you do has to start with you FIRST. This is not about being narcissistic, self-absorbed, or selfish; it is about prioritizing your health, your love for yourself, and your desire to be a responsible adult.

"Our capacity for self-love filters our experience of the world," says Alexandra Katehakis, PhD, Clinical Director of Center for Healthy Sex and author of *Erotic Intelligence.* This is very important to understand. Oftentimes, people that have problems recognizing their self-worth take things too personally and often perceive them in a negative way. As Katehakis says, "the more self-love we practice, the more we love others." Please, practice self-love and be patient with yourself and your partner. Grow your self-esteem and do not take things personally, I'm sure you want to get close to each other but do not know how.

Start with awareness—awareness of yourself, your body, and your genitalia. Sex is what you do, behavior and acts, which are performed with the body. So, it is through your body that you express and act out your sexual desires, your sexual thoughts, and your sexuality. Masturbation is an important activity in order to be aware of your sexual needs and how your body works. It is part of being healthy and having a satisfying sex life.

Well-known American sexologist, biologist, and outstanding researcher Dr. Alfred Kinsey, who founded the Institute for Sex Research at Indiana University in 1947, known as the Kinsey Institute, reported that women who masturbated before marriage had a much better likelihood of achieving orgasms during sexual activities with their partners.

Moreover, sex therapist Louanne Cole Weston, PhD, author of *Sex Matters*, affirms that "masturbation helps with an imbalance and helps couples avoid being coerced up or down in frequency by their partner. It's an aid to a relationship over the long haul." Planned Parenthood, a national organization for sexual and reproductive health, states that "it's totally normal to masturbate (touch yourself for sexual pleasure) whether you're sexually active with other people or not. Masturbation even has health benefits, like reducing stress... Masturbation can actually be good for your health, both mentally and physically. And it's pretty much the safest sex out there—there's no risk of getting pregnant or getting an STD."

We can see through the past and present researches that masturbation, or solo sex, can not only improve your relationship and sex life, but also can improve your overall health. Everyone is different, and even though we all need exercise, nutrition, sleep, rest, love, and orgasms, different bodies require these things differently. Be conscious about what your body (your only vehicle) needs and get to know your preferences to be as healthy as possible to *make love 365 times a year.* Ask yourself:

▶ What kind of food will help me create a healthier body? It is up to you to find out what is good for your body's well-being. It is not about satisfying your gluttony with tasty food but nourishing your body with nutritious food.

▶ What kind of exercises are good and appropriate for me to strengthen my muscle and bones? What activities can I do to help my body get healthier? It is up to you, too.

▶ What kind of sexual activities do I prefer? What do I like sexually? What turns me on? What turns me off? How many orgasms do I need per week/month?

When thinking of your body as the vehicle, think that you want a vehicle that works properly. The better the car, the better the drive will be. The better you treat your body, the better it will function or respond. And, just as you maintain your car, you must maintain your body. As you would get your oil changed, put gas in the car, and fill the tires with air, you must service your body with water, food, sleep, rest, and orgasms for good functioning! Otherwise, how will your body work properly if you do not treat it well?

We all need a healthy sexual mindset and a healthy body (as healthy as possible) to *make love 365 times a year.* I have found that the following four areas have a tremendous impact on sexual satisfaction. Please pay attention to these areas to start shaping your lifestyle and improving your sex life:

1. Self-esteem, self-image, self-worth
2. What you eat: nutritious food and plenty of water
3. Exercise, rest, and fun
4. Sexual health: it is not just about overcoming your sexual problems but being able to experience joy and sexual pleasure.

When Sarah and Frank were not taking care of themselves, they were not taking care of their sex life, either. At the end of our sessions, I warned them that, if they were not willing to change their unhealthy lifestyle now, they would soon stop having sex completely and grow apart into roommates. It was not too late for them, it is never too late if you dare to improve things, and they did! They took a step forward and started changing their health habits for good.

They ended up changing their lifestyle completely, and as result of this change, they started enjoying their sex life again and making love more often! It was not easy, but it was possible! Now you know my Sex Secret #2: A Healthy Lifestyle—that starts with you.

Remember, your body is an important variable—the physical element—to *make love 365 times a year.* Now, let's work on getting the best of your body—the only "vehicle" you have.

Please observe Sarah's and Frank's Lovemaking Wheel. Pay attention to the 2ⁿᵈ area: a healthy lifestyle. In their Lovemaking Wheels, it is very clear that Sex Secret #2 is missing.

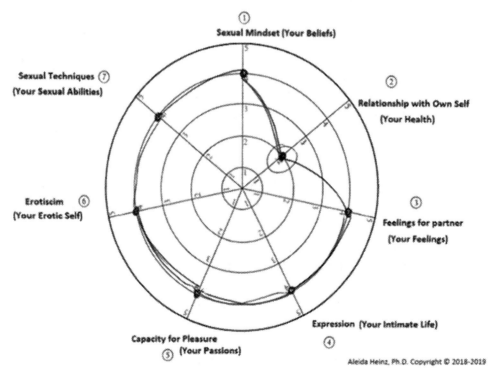

Sarah's Lovemaking Wheel. Wheel #3

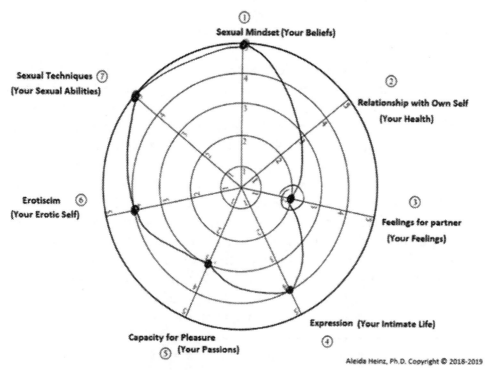

Frank's Lovemaking Wheel. Wheel #4

My hope is that by reading the following parts, you understand the importance of improving your health through a good, healthy lifestyle in order to *make love 365 times a year.*

Part II: A Healthy Lifestyle for a Healthy Sex Life

We cannot choose where to be born or how to grow up, but we can choose how to live our lives as adults. It is not about money but about choices. The actions we choose and the decisions we make every day determine our lifestyle. Let's begin by understanding what a lifestyle is. First, differentiate the activities outside of your routine, those that you put conscious effort into doing in; and then the activities you do normally as a way of living, as part of your routine. The first group of activities is based on effort. You should concentrate on doing them, focus, and plan them. The second group, the routine, are effortless actions—actions without much effort—that you can easily do without much work or thought.

For example, a person with no healthy habits who is trying to lose weight may diet hard or try to walk some set number of miles a day with a great deal of effort to reach the goal. These are conscious activities this person must do outside of their routine. The diet or the walking strategy are being done with effort in a conscious way—concentration, focus, and plan. However, if this person already has a lifestyle that involves healthy eating and exercise as part of his/her routine, then, losing weight would be much easier and take much less effort since these activities are already part of daily life—a lifestyle.

In my own life, for instance, I have created a lifestyle where I do not eat many carbs, any sugar, or any meat. Instead, I eat green salads and vegetables most days. By eating this way for so long, I have created a lifestyle where eating green salads and avoiding sugar is now effortless, it's part of my everyday eating, so I don't suffer when I will eat salads instead of pizza, for instance. This is only one aspect of life. What about the other aspects? Same thing! Effort-based vs. effortless activities. Effortless activities are your routine, the familiar things you do daily. Your routine involves different aspects of your life and that is your lifestyle: the way you do things unconsciously—can be good for your health or very bad. Consider what you do and how you do it to evaluate if you need to improve. Remember habits. Habits shape your lifestyle.

I share the view of professor of integrative medicine in neurological surgery at Weill Cornell Medical Center and founder and director of PATH (Place for Achieving Total Health) Medical center, Dr. Eric R. Braverman, MD, author of *Younger (Thinner) You Diet and Younger Sexier You*, that "it's natural to be unhappy about certain aspects of your life from time to time, especially if you are focused on your weight. But when you are unhappy about every aspect of your life, it may be time to get professional help." Be aware that your lifestyle is an expression of yourself, as American clinical psychologist and Nevada Foundation Professor in the Behavior Analysis program at the University of Nevada, Steven C. Hayes, PhD, says: "Expressions of what you care about, they profoundly inform what you pursue day to day, year to year. In so doing, they fundamentally shape the trajectory of your life."

It reflects not only who you are, but what you want out of life. It is the manifestation of how you have decided to live your life. You are doing things every day, in every aspect: mentally, emotionally, spiritually, physically, and sexually. How are you feeling and doing in each of these aspects? Are you improving? Are you growing? A healthy lifestyle is a healthy way of living and relating to others that will allow your constant improvement and growth.

So, let's create a healthy lifestyle for a fantastic sex life. But how?

Remember Sex Secret #1: your sexual mindset, where I talked about crafting habits. By consciously creating healthy habits, you will eventually be able to mold them into an unconscious healthy lifestyle. Therefore, habits form your lifestyle and can create an unhealthy or healthy lifestyle. Your lifestyle is up to your level of awareness!

The point is that you need healthy habits in every area of your life. These habits will become behaviors that will improve you in every sense—physically, mentally, emotionally, spiritually, and sexually. Therefore, anything you do regularly, easily, effortless, and unconsciously as part of your routine needs to make you better, until you become the BEST version of yourself.

Always keep in mind that your habits, good or bad, create your lifestyle. So, if most of your habits are good and healthy, your lifestyle will be too! Any positive habits not only help you but your relationship as well. When you care for yourself first through exercising, healthy eating, and proper sleep, as well as caring for your sexuality; that is, your whole body, it maximizes your potential in your everyday life. So, you become your best you, you can reach out to others and have the best relationships possible with them. This, of course, includes your partner!

You need to feel good, sexy, and energetic for a satisfying sex life. Remember Sarah and Frank—they both lacked a healthy lifestyle, and therefore had a poor sex life. Now, you need to add life to your sex life, you must see your sexuality as an essential element in your lifestyle—part of your life and well-being.

To some people, this might sound too difficult, especially if they have unhealthy habits that include poor nutrition, no exercise, bad sleeping, and dysfunctional relationships. The concept of having a healthy lifestyle sounds great in theory, but how can you achieve it? Again, think back to Chapter 1—by working first on your mindsets. You first have to change the way you view and treat your body. You must change your mindset about the importance of your body to overcome unhealthy bodily habits.

Therefore, I started with mindset first. Not only do you need to have a sexual mindset, but also a mindset that allows you to keep healthy habits to keep healthy body and healthy genitals. If you commit yourself to a better lifestyle, then you may find the time, tools, and the energy to go ahead and do it. Be patient and committed to a healthy lifestyle. The rest will follow.

Belief and Behavior

1. BELIEF: Your mindset must be pro-healthy habits. If you believe that exercise, nutrition, sleep, stress reduction, orgasm, and fun are all great for your overall health, then you will be motivated to experience them. Believe in yourself, believe in your partner—the one you love and loves you—believe in the process, and believe that you can do it!

2. BEHAVIORS: When you believe you can do it; you do! You will take action and move forward to create the love life you want. Actions are behaviors, a requirement to form habits: do something repeatedly, act and be consistent and persevering until it is easy to do so. Avoid overthinking. I know that at the beginning you will need to make a great effort but then you won't have to make so much effort, believe me, and believe in you!

These two "B" steps—belief and behavior—apply to everything you might do: sports, business, love, etc. And they apply to everyone regardless of age, social status, culture, health conditions, gender, or education. Achieving your goals is about discipline and commitment. Dr. Beecham, from Chapter 1, says, "believing that you will do well keeps your mind free from distractions and anxious thoughts, leaving you with a quiet mind (not thinking) that leads to a great performance (behavior)…and frees your mind to focus on the here and now."

Set rituals and healthy habits today, here and now—don't put it off! Believe in them and act. The worst thing you can do is to say, I'll start it later, or I'll wait for such and such a time. What is wrong with now? Even small changes can have powerful impacts, such as kissing your partner every morning when you wake up, walking every day, smiling frequently, or going to bed earlier alongside your partner.

A healthy lifestyle will allow you to enjoy more your love life. Part of a healthy lifestyle are good love habits—things you do effortlessly and naturally do to keep the "fire" in your relationship. You together form these habits over time. Be aware of them. Make sure they are positive and bring them closer, and not negative and keep them away. Start forming new love habits today. Remember, it's never too late!

Love habits are key to maintain your love life in shape. A loving, happy love life is built out of many daily behaviors and actions—love habits—that keep the connection and the passion alive between you and your partner.

I fought and struggled to create my own healthy lifestyle long ago. As I got older and busier, it would have been easy to give up. But because I created good habits early on, now in my almost 55s I have a healthy lifestyle that allows me to enjoy an active and fulfilling sex life. Pedro and I *make love 365 times a year* and will keep doing it, as long as we are alive and committed to growth and connection—in our own way. I do what I preach!

Begin your days with healthy morning routine, such as thoughts of gratitude, a smile, a kiss, water, some stretching, a healthy breakfast, and lovemaking—there's nothing like morning sex to set your day. Then follow the other daily stuff, such as work, chores, exercise, family time, etc. Set your own morning routine, according to your needs, to set the tone of your day. If you feel positive and optimistic in the morning, you may feel good or better for the rest of the day, with a strong immune system, even in difficult times.

Researchers have found that a healthy lifestyle is based on many factors. In my opinion, the following thirteen habits are the main factors you need to work on for a great and healthy lifestyle. The one you deserve! The thirteen healthy habits are:

1. Time management: Time is precious! It is an invaluable resource we all have, but not all appreciate it. Steve Jobs says: "My favorite things in life don't cost any money. It's really clear that the most precious resource we all have is time." The first thing to enjoy the benefits of a healthy lifestyle is to control your time to balance your life, regardless of external circumstances. In my practice, I constantly receive calls from people who claim their sex life and relationships are falling apart, but when I try to set an appointment with them, they say they don't have time! How will you fix or improve yourself or your relationship if you can't commit time to do so? You must create a balance.

Many people claim they work so much that they are just too tired for their partners and they don't have time to relax and enjoy each other, but they want to have a happy relationship. How? It's like saying—you can't stop for gas because you don't have time, but if the tank runs empty, what will you do? If your relationship and your sex life are important to you, then find the time to work on them. Beecham remain us that "everyone has the same amount of time, but successful people value their time more, and thus they are more efficient."

Learn to be more efficient in the areas of your life you care most about. What are those areas? Are you giving them time? Do you want to *make love 365 times a year*?

Everyone has twenty-four hours in a day. The key is to manage which activities you do in these 24 hours. You must be wise with your time to create your own healthy lifestyle. Once you own your time, you can prioritize the other twelve items on the list. Become aware of your priorities! You cannot accomplish anything if your priorities are not in line with your goals. If you can't put your sex life first, then it will be difficult to *make love 365 times a year...*

2. Stress Control: Nowadays, almost everyone says they are stressed; it seems to be "normal." But stress control doesn't mean not having problems; it means facing problems strategically and *controlling your reactions* to them. That is, reacting proactively so as not to have to overload generating stress. It is we who produce stress, not our problems. Problems are there for us to learn and keep growing, not for us to stress out.

Remember the lesson from Chapter 1: we can't control the outside world. But we can control how we react to the challenges that come our way. According to Braverman, "hormonal imbalances can start even earlier (before menopause) when brain stress is high." Arianna Huffington wisely advises in her posts that "you can achieve everything without having to lose your health, and your relationship and what matters to you." It is a very wise advice, and so it is that stress can ruin your sex life as it reduces pleasure, sexual desire, interest in sex, genital response, and your overall sexual functioning greatly.

3. Be exposed to nature: Studies show that interaction with nature, like sunlight exposure, barefoot contact with the ground, breathing fresh air, and feeling ocean and river water, can lift your mood and improve your health. Natural sunlight is a great source of vitamin D, serotonin, and metabolism-boosting—nutrients for a healthy body. In fact, researchers have shown that a lack of vitamin D is linked to numerous signs of aging.

Also, sunlight is known to increase your body's production of testosterone and serotonin, so if you don't get enough sun, your hormone levels may drop, making you feel moody and depressed.

4. Have a strong social network: Online in times of crisis and real-life group of friends and family. It is important to talk to people for fun and in times of need—a support net. While you may use the Internet or phone to maintain these contacts, make sure you are having quality time and face-to-face interactions with those who matter, especially with your partner! I recommend that you and your partner make friends together, not as individuals but as a couple, to spend some fun time together—as a couple.

5. Be relaxed and have fun: Any activities that please you are important, no matter how small. Being able to experience pleasure—even small pleasures—is fundamental for a healthy and fulfilling sex life. I talk in more in depth about pleasure in Chapter 5.

6. Ensure meaning in your life: What are you doing in your daily life? What are your intentions? What are your goals in life? Meaning may be produced through your career, a job, or a hobby—any way that you can create something and give something positive back into the world. Be aware of the meaning of your daily actions. "The why" of your actions is important to understand before you act. Beecham says, "a big part of success training involves truly understanding why you are doing what you are doing, how to do it, and what it is you are doing."

7. Stay away from destructive habits: To *make love 365 times a year,* staying away from bad habits is essential! Bad habits are things that you do that will not help you improve or grow, on the contrary, they harm you, and can negatively affect your love life. For example, the vice or bad habit of smoking. As I always say, "the worst enemy of the penis, and your health, is certainly cigarettes." According to medical expert Dr. Chris Iliades, MD, who has 20 years of experience in clinical medicine and clinical research, "smoking is the biggest cause of erectile dysfunction. That's because maintaining an erection requires a healthy blood supply, and nicotine causes your blood vessels to contract, which

causes the penis to shrink. The longer you're a smoker, the more difficult it is to treat or reverse erectile dysfunction."

Also, any kind of drug, including marijuana and excessive amounts of alcohol, can be detrimental to your sexual health. According to the NuMale Medical Center, "marijuana use has been shown to lower testosterone levels, and low-T can contribute to ED. Marijuana use has also been associated with orgasm-related problems (both premature ejaculation and inability to achieve orgasm)." Likewise, a 2010 study published in the Journal European Urology found that marijuana may contribute to ED by inhibiting the nervous system response that causes an erection in the first place.

Addictions of any kind can make you a slave by controlling your behavior and your free will. Habits can be positive and good, or negative and bad. Bad habits prevent good sexual functioning and deteriorate your brain, your body, your health, your sex life, and your relationships. Stay away from negative habits! I know you can do it, if you really want to *make love 365 times a year*!

8. Be in touch with your emotions: You need to learn to be assertive with your emotions—I don't mean be explosive and angry—I mean you shouldn't repress yourself, nor should you overreact. Express how you are feeling, especially to your partner. Validate your own emotions and express them without reacting or acting upon them. Talk about your emotions to your partner, it is important. Learning to recognize and express your feelings is fundamental in the formation of intimacy. I have dedicated the next chapter (Chapter 3) to the importance of your feelings in a pleasurable sex life. Make expressing your feelings a positive habit in your life.

9. Communicate with those in your life: This is especially true with your partner. You need someone you can be yourself with, and who better than your partner to fill that need? Communication is the key to intimacy. Be sure to communicate more! I have also dedicated a whole chapter to the subject of communication (Chapter 4).

10. Self-acceptance: Self-acceptance is one of the fundamentals of self-esteem. You should have strong high self-esteem (love for yourself) in order to be loved and make love. Working to improve your

self-esteem—and partner's—will have a great impact on how you perceive each other, the world, and your love life. It is hard or almost impossible to enjoy a fulfilling sex life while having poor self-esteem. Remember, your perception affects satisfaction.

11. Safe living: Safety is important. This means to be as safe as possible in your own space. Even if it is just a room or a small area, you need to feel safe to grow and have a pleasant time. One of the requirements for a healthy sexuality is safety.

12. Keep a healthy body: Nutrition, exercise, sleep, downtime, orgasms, affection, and fun are fundamental requirements to enjoy life and keep a strong immune system, so essential these days. Keep this in mind!

13. Keep a healthy sex life: Clinical sexologist, sexuality educator, and a pioneer of sex coaching, Dr. Patti Britton, says: "It's no secret that a healthy sex life is essential for happy, long-lasting relationships." Feel good and better about yourself, about your partner, about sex, and about your love life. This is the foundation for a healthy sex life: a healthy you! Make *lovemaking* a healthy love habit so that making love will be part of your daily life. Something special that you will do every day...

There are many healthy lifestyles that will help everyone, but you must know your own body and the type of life you want to know what will work best for you. Therefore, the development of your unique lifestyle is important. Make it as healthy as possible!

Part III: A Healthy Body for Better Sex

Remember the GPS and the car analogy? The GPS can't do anything by itself without a car, but without the GPS, the car can drive but might get lost. A healthy brain and positive mind (GPS) are needed to "drive" your body (the car). If you have a car in good condition, regardless of the brand, model or year, it can drive you anywhere as long as it's guided by a workable GPS. The same is true for your body. If your body is in good condition, regardless of age, race, or culture, it can take you anywhere you want to—in bed or out of bed—guided by a positive sexual mindset.

But without a functional body; that is, with a body in a precarious condition, you can't go very far even with an excellent mindset. Your mind may be incapable of fully fulfilling its task. If your body—your car—is in the best possible condition, you will be able to enact the desires of your mind. Keep in mind that your sexual mind—not your body—is the one that leads, and it is the most powerful force you have to enjoy sexual pleasures.

Studies have shown a correlation between how you feel about yourself and sexual satisfaction. Recent studies indicate that moderate weight loss through healthy eating can significantly improve your sex life and satisfaction. As Braverman in *Younger (Thinner) your Diet* points out, "even moderate weight loss results in significant improvements in sexual functioning and satisfaction. And those who regularly exercise have higher levels of desire and enhanced ability to achieve orgasm." Similarly, other studies have shown that people who exercise regularly and eat nutritionally have higher sexual desire and a greater ability to get aroused and experience orgasm.

Sounds great, right? The better you feel, the better your sex life will be! Isn't that what we want? So, how do you keep a healthy body throughout your whole life to *make love 365 times a year*?

Let's take a look at your life right now. How healthy is your diet? Your diet is the #1 element for a healthy body. As I once read, 70% of your health is diet and 30% is exercise. The healthier a person eats, the better their sex life will be…and the more active and pleasant your sex life is, the healthier your diet will be! It is a true catch-22. Do you know why?

According to a report by the Archives of General Psychiatry Journal, poor diet and excess weight literally clutter the brain, causing all kinds of issues, including sexual problems. In other words, great sex comes from a healthy brain, and a healthy brain comes from a healthy diet! No doubt about it! As we get older, men and women both produce less and less of the "big three" sex hormones: estrogen, progesterone, and testosterone, making us feel less sexy and sexually motivated. So, nutrition is key for keeping your hormones in balance to keep your body as healthy as possible.

Now, different bodies have diverse needs; that is, different instructions for care, just like different cars have different manuals. But some care is universal—you must put fuel in any car, rotate the tires, and change the oil—and some body care is universal as well: you must drink water, get nutrients, move your body, and sleep.

These four-universal musts—water, nutrients, movement, sleep—are requisite for everyone who wants to keep a healthy body, despite their age, gender, cultural background, economic status, or any other factors. These things are vital for ANYONE on Earth! Let's explore these universal musts: A) Nutritious Eating and Water. B) Sleep and Rest. C) Regular Exercise—movement.

A. Nutritious Eating and Water: Nutrition is not my specialty. I am not a nutritionist or health coach, so the purpose of this section is not to tell you what or how to eat, but to explore the role food plays in your sexuality and how nutrition is essential for great sex, especially to *make love 365 times a year.* Eating well is very important, more than we can imagine. After water, nutrition is the main element for a healthy body. Doctors agree that without healthy eating, exercise and proper sleep won't have much of an impact on helping you create a healthy body.

But what does healthy eating have to do with sex? My first rule of great sex: whatever is good for your heart is good for your genitals! If something is good for your heart, it's good for your penis or vulva, too; they are dependent on blood flow just like your heart. Too much bad food and bad fats create vascular problems and keep blood from easily getting into your genitals—especially your penis, if you are a man.

Think of it like dust in an air vent. Keep restricting the passage with dust—or bad fats—and nothing else can pass through. For example, we know that blockages of blood vessels due to high-fat, high-cholesterol diets are not restricted to the heart's coronaries. The arteries that supply blood to the penis clog up, too, as mentioned in the Practical Encyclopedia of Sex and Health.

Documentary filmmaker Kip Andersen speaks in his book and documentary *What The Health*, about the Oxford study which advises that eating meat four times a week increases your cancer risk by 42%. Not good for an active sex life! Dr. Linda De Villers, PhD, author of *Simple Sexy Food*, recommends a great diversity of healthy food for fostering your libido. De Villers says that she wrote her book "to help you enjoy the remarkable relationship between food and sex."

Dr. Steven Gundry, MD—mentioned in the introduction—director of the International Heart and Lung Institute in Palm Springs, and the founder and director of the Center for Restorative Medicine, reminds us to eat plenty of greens daily for a healthy body, and even to reverse certain illnesses. As Gundry says in *The Longevity Paradox*: "The idea that heart disease is not an inevitability, and that it can actually be reversed without surgery or medication, goes against everything I once believed as a heart surgeon and cardiologist... But what if I told you that just about everything you've ever been told about heart disease is dead wrong? Not only about the heart but also about our entire bodies and our health in general."

Food plays an important role in sex, and one example is the correlation between GABA (a brain chemical) and orgasm. As mentioned by Braverman, "orgasm is controlled by our levels of GABA. If GABA becomes depleted, you can't relax or let go, and hence, you can't have an orgasm." So, consuming food that boosts GABA production, like kale and spinach, is essential for great sex as well. I eat them every day. Why not start today?

What about sexual desire? What does food have to do with it? The answer: A LOT!

Braverman affirms that "desire is created in the brain by dopamine, when you are low on dopamine your energy for and interest in sex wanes. So, boosting dopamine production is essential as well, and you can do that by cutting out as many sugary foods and processed simple carbs from your diet as possible."

Then, nutrition is one of the big keys to great sex, right?

A study published in a psychopharmacology journal, by S. Brody & R. Preut, shows that ascorbic acid (vitamin C) has many functions. It is important for healthy sexuality through mechanisms such as the reduction of anxiety and stress, the modulation of brain dopaminergic and noradrenergic activities, cardiovascular support, and oxytocin secretion. Poor nutrition affects your entire body in the same way that poor maintenance deteriorates your vehicle, like putting contaminated gas in your car. The car will run, but it won't work well. And after a time, problems will arise—maybe not at first, but eventually you will lack energy and finally break down. Creating those healthy habits early on will keep you from breaking down later in life!

A healthy diet will lead to healthier sex for so many reasons, as explained before. Think about this for a second: How do you feel when you lose weight, eat clean, and exercise? Do you feel energized and sexy? Because I do! I feel great when I discipline myself by eating good foods, drinking plenty of water, and working out daily, regardless of problems or external factors around me.

As a sexologist, I help people develop fulfilling relationships, which include sexual satisfaction. Low or no desire for sex—the most common of sexual problems among women and men—can be triggered by medical conditions or hormone imbalance. However, for a lot of women, a big libido killer is their own self-image, or self-esteem, and their own relationships. Hormonal imbalance can have a lot to do with what you eat, and what you eat affects your self-image. You might be unhappy sexually simply because you are not eating well, and likewise, you feel tired, stressed out, too fat or too thin, and depressed.

The good news is that you can live fully and have a better sex life all by eating healthy, in addition to the other factors I will show you later. And, you don't have to make radical changes to improve your diet. Start small, step by step. Try to avoid eating your kid's snacks, your partner's dinner, and all the garbage that tastes so good. Simply cut out putting sugar in your coffee, drink more water, be sure to eat a healthy breakfast, and turn down dessert when eating out. And with the Internet as a cookbook, it is easier than ever to find healthy alternatives to our favorite meals! See where that begins to lead you.

And yes, drink more water! Don't forget to drink plenty of water! Remember how I always start my day with almost a liter of water! This is important to restore your metabolism, which will give you more energy. Energy keeps your body alive and helps move your body—this will lead to desire! Water is also crucial to great sex! It contributes to your good blood flow, since blood is 94% water and you need fluid blood to fill your sex organs. A lack of water makes your blood too thick. Imagine your blood like a smoothie. If you only put in fruit, it's too thick to move through the straw. You have to add juice—or in your case, water—to let it flow easier.

Many health professionals, coaches, and trainers highly recommend eating protein and green shakes at your daily breakfast to start the day off with mental alertness and energy, balanced blood sugar, proper cortisol levels, and to help you snack less. It seems that eating protein early in the day affects gastrointestinal hormones, which signal the brain to adjust appetite and satiety. One study found that after a protein meal, there was a significant drop in ghrelin (a hunger-stimulating hormone) and an elevation in PYY (a satiety-stimulating hormone). Therefore, protein to start the day may be the way to go…of course, after morning lovemaking!

Please remember that there are no magic pills for great sex, for being healthy, staying sexy, or making love. The truth is, you and only you have the power to create magic in your life, especially in your sex life, if you pay attention to your body. Listen to your body! The real aphrodisiacs, beside a sexy partner, are good foods full of nutrients that allow optimal sexual functioning. Once you've begun eating healthy, everything else will follow.

B. Sleep and Rest: We all know we need to sleep. But how does this relate to sex? Remember, you only have one unique vehicle, your body. It needs both rest and proper sleep. Rest and sleep are different activities in which the body restores all its functions, but in different ways. Rest is mainly body inactivity, in which the mind can be calm and quiet, producing relaxation. It is about giving your body and mind a break, or time-out, to recharge them. On the other hand, sleep is the shutdown of body and mind so that the brain can refresh, repair, or regenerate its cells by going into the stages of sleep: REM and non-REM sleep.

According to the National Sleep Foundation, "resting with your eyes closed can calm your mind, give at least some of your neurons a break, and let your muscles and organs relax. It can also reduce stress, improve your mood, and increase alertness, mental clarity, creativity, and motivation... It's only in the deeper stages of slumber that you get a substantial cognitive boost, increase your ability to remember new information, repair or regenerate cells themselves, and the release of growth hormone and other hormones."

You may wonder how much rest and sleep you need—and what about sex? Experts in the field say that the average person needs deep, uninterrupted sleep for 7 to 8 hours a day. During deep, uninterrupted sleep, your brain is experiencing slower wave lengths and rapid eye movements. These help your vitals and restore your bodily functions. Shelly Ibach, CEO and president of Sleep Number and Thrive Sleep Editor refers to sleep as "universal" and says that "we all need it. But how we achieve quality sleep is individualized."

Most importantly, serotonin is produced while you sleep. This is a hormone that raises your mood, so you are calm and tranquil during the day. It also lowers your desire for sugar (overconsumption of which will lead to the problems I discussed above) and helps you with anxiety. When you get less sleep, you get less serotonin, which is considered a pleasure hormone, serotonin will give you a good calm mood which can lead to sex. In addition, Dr. Mitchel F. Roizen, MD has proven that if you get less sleep than you need, you're at an "increased risk of a heart attack." When your body resets during sleep, your heart and arteries get younger and healthier, which is great for your genitals.

Therefore, "your body needs both sleep and rest...the important thing is to give your mind and body a chance to recover and recharge when you're feeling out of steam," as the National Sleep Foundation recommends.

Want even better sleep?

Studies have shown that these benefits increase if you *sleep naked.* Sleeping naked lower your body temperature, which boosts metabolism and improves blood circulation, sperm quality, skin, and genital health. Studies show that optimal sleep happens when your bedroom is between 60 and 68 degrees. Anything above 70 will cause the body to overheat and make you wake up. Lowering your body temperature by being naked helps activate brown fat—a type of fat that helps regulate your body temperature by generating heat. Research shows that people with higher levels of brown fat have faster resting metabolic rates, better blood sugar control, and higher insulin sensitivity. In one study, sleeping in a chilled room doubled the amount of brown fat participants produced. So, you're also raising your metabolism by sleeping naked!

For men, sleeping naked also elevates sperm count! Testicles are designed to keep sperm at a temperature just slightly below core body temperature. Underwear that bunches the testicles close to the body may, therefore, reduce sperm quality and affect a man's fertility. In women, sleeping without underwear can lower the risk of yeast infections because warm, moist environments most often cause them. And, without pajamas, your blood flow is less restricted, so your genitals may be ready for morning sex! Your sex life will benefit as well! Sleeping naked doesn't necessarily lead to morning sex, but it increases your skin-to-skin contact with your partner, raising the hormone oxytocin.

Oxytocin promotes feelings of attachment and emotional closeness, making you both feel connected through the day, and strengthening your bonds. Multiple studies have shown the relationship between oxytocin, vasopressin hormones (released by skin-to-skin contact in the mornings) and fidelity. So, now you know that sleeping naked is great for your health, your sex life, and your relationship! This simple habit benefits not only your entire body, but your love life as well! Turn it into a love habit! Moreover, there is nothing more effective than sex to sleep well and relieve pain. Sex releases endorphins and corticosteroids, which can help relieve pain. Painkillers, on the other hand, may delay orgasm and be addictive.

   C. Regular Exercise—movement: There is a proven link between sex and exercise. When you exercise, the brain immediately produces *endorphins* that stimulate the release of sex hormones. I always wait for that moment! Even if I'm tired, I remind myself that the endorphins will kick in and help me to start working out and get in the mood. Sure enough, in five to ten minutes, I feel different. These hormones reduce your heart rate, improve digestion, lower blood pressure and cortisol levels, and relax the body: in other words, it puts you in the best condition to have sex.

A 2008 study conducted at Florida Atlantic University found that men and women who exercised frequently were more likely to rate themselves higher regarding sexual performance and sexual desirability. Studies have also shown that women who frequently exercise become aroused more quickly and are able to orgasm faster and experience it more intensely.

Stress management is fundamental to lower cortisol levels in order to enjoy a better sex life! Low levels relax your body, which equals great sex! So, beyond making you look sexier and stronger, exercise will lead to increased sex hormones, and lower blood pressure and cortisol levels. This lower blood pressure will help blood flow levels, which, as we discussed with healthy eating, will help your genitals be healthier, too. There are only benefits to exercise!

Know that when I say exercise, I mean some kind of physical movement. You don't have to become a bodybuilder, an athlete, or a bikini fitness model! Just make sure you are moving your whole body daily. This depends on your own physical restrictions, age, and other limitations, so find what works best for you—but do it! It is recommended to exercise at least 15 to 30 minutes per day. Strength training is also recommended, it increases levels of growth hormone, which contributes to spikes in testosterone. Including strength training, like weight training, in your routine two or three times per week, has been shown to improve sexual functioning.

In my case, I have had two fractures—wrist and ankle—plus knee surgery. I'm careful, but I do exercise almost every day, to the best of my ability. No excuses! I don't run on the treadmill but walk or spin intensely and concentrate more on my abs and legs. Go little by little to get stronger and find what works best for you. For some, this might be swimming, for others an aerobics class—and there are always those who love to run! The key is to listen to your body and keep moving to *make love 365 times a year!*

"Add more physical activity to every part of your day... One of my favorite forms of exercise for increasing GABA (the brain chemical needed for relaxation) is Pilates," says Braverman, and I agree! I love Pilates, yoga, ballet, and especially spinning. Braverman also advises that "physical movement—whether aerobic or anaerobic—helps to reset the brain and release serotonin. Resolution is related to serotonin. If serotonin becomes depleted, your timing is off. You're either coming 'to the party' too early or too late."

Moreover, S.S. Curry, PhD, acknowledges that "a true exercise always brings some specific part (of your body) into action…Never regard your exercise as merely physical. All training is an action of the mind. It just may manifest itself in a physical direction." It is very important to understand that exercising the body is not only important to keep you in good shape, but to be your very best. I share the findings of Beecham: "for humans to be at their best, we need to do physically strenuous activities (which release endorphin) and to complete tasks and have a sense of accomplishment (which release dopamine). We cannot be our best self unless we live our life this way." Being your best self also means being sexually happy and fulfilled.

Think about all the possibilities for your body. Remember your healthy lifestyle—a large part of a healthy lifestyle is time management. It's important to find time to exercise! This will help your mind, and your body gets in shape to *make love 365 times a year.*

The Sex Muscle

Now, let's talk about your sex muscle! The pubococcygeal (PC) muscles provide support to the pelvic floor, holding your organs in place. By strengthening your PC muscles, you will strengthen and support your sexual functioning in many ways. The PC muscles also provide support to urethra, bladder, and bowel. Men, as well as women, need to strengthen the PC muscles, our sex muscles, to enjoy *making love 356 times a year.*

How? By training your PC through the exercise known as Kegels. The best and only way to keep your PC healthy and strong is through Kegels. There are specific exercises to do Kegels that work for both females and males. Kegels, or PC exercises, benefit women by helping them to feel stronger orgasms and tighten their vaginal walls. They benefit men by helping them to sustain longer and stronger erections, and to control ejaculation: not too fast and not too slow. Also, both men and women can learn to use their strengthened PC muscles for power pumping in sex play.

The PC Exercise

Locate your PC muscle, on the pelvic floor, by stopping and starting the flow of urine. Do it ONLY ONCE, just to identify your PC muscles. Then, never use that technique again when you want to urinate, in other words, with a full bladder. Do it only with an empty bladder.

Use the following pattern for daily practice with your empty bladder:

A. Locate the muscle and squeeze it tightly for two to five seconds. Count one, two...five to time your hold.
B. Release it for one second.
C. Repeat this exercise ten times, three times a day, for the first two weeks, for a total of 30 daily repetitions to start with. Then, increase to 20 times, three times a day, and so on to reach 100 per day or for 10 minutes a day. Make sure to rest for 20 seconds between repetitions. Go slow!
D. Do this EVERY day for three weeks to start with, then do it as a habit, a long-term behavior—always! You will find a marked positive change in your sex life. Your penis will stay harder, longer; you will feel your orgasms more powerfully (both men and women) and feel more confident in bed.

After three weeks of regular PC or Kegel exercises, women report tighter vaginas and more intense orgasms. Men have firmer and harder erections. Do your PC exercises as part of your lifestyle to improve and maintain your sex muscle, keeping it in good shape and ready for sex.

Both sexes can use their PC muscles effectively during sexual intercourse. In one ancient sexual secret technique, named Pompoirpower, the female flexes her muscles around the penis (or pumps it) making him feel like she is sucking his penis to ejaculation. Remember, sex is something you do with your body, including your genitals. This exercise is for your genitals! You must have functioning body and genitals to have a functioning sex life. You want a vivid and awake body for a passionate sex life.

Sexuality has to be turned on, just like you would turn on the car. You can't go anywhere with the car off! Once you're turned on, then you can direct your body to go in the direction you want to go. This is what I mean by properly functioning. When you are not responding at all, or not being turned on, you probably think it may be a problem, a sexual problem. If the car isn't switching on, it's having trouble responding, it needs to be turned on, right? Other problems can be responding too fast—Rapid Ejaculation— or too slow—Delayed Ejaculation, for instance. If the GPS is okay, but the vehicle is not, then you have a problem, don't you?

Don't think of sexual problems as right or wrong, or good or bad; just think about whether your body is functioning according to your needs and desires. Just as your car not starting would not be a moral issue, neither is your body's inability to respond to sexual stimuli. We just need to explore what prevents your body from responding, with delicacy and compassion. On many occasions, the desires of the mind and heart do not match the genital response, and vice versa. This should not be a problem since the important thing is intention and desire. There are several ways to assist the body for good response.

The key is to listen to your body. Every vehicle is different and needs different care. The most important thing you can do is find out what helps you and makes you feel the best for a good sexual response. While there are differences for every person, being mindful of nutritious eating, drinking enough water, sleep and rest, and exercise are part of a healthy lifestyle. With these elements for your health, you open the door to all possibilities, and to *make love 365 times a year.*

And remember—what may work for one body may not work for another. That is why knowing yourself first, having the capacity to adapt to different stages of life with flexibility, and keeping healthy habits in place, are so important.

Keep going! The only failure is to quit…

Part IV: Sexual Health

I have been talking about the importance of a healthy lifestyle in which nutrition, exercise, and sleep are fundamental to keep your body in good physical condition. Now, a crucial component of your overall health is your sexual health. There is no such thing as being healthy without being sexually healthy as well.

Studies have found that about 94% of people consider that being sexually healthy enriches their quality of life. There are plenty studies that show the multiple benefits of healthy sex. For instance, according to Dr. Dominguez-Bali, MD at Miami Center for Obstetrics, Gynecology & Human Sexuality, "orgasms benefit the circulatory, neural, muscular, articular, hormonal as well as the Genito-urinary system." So, to be truly healthy, your sexual health must also be taken care of. This doesn't just mean having healthy genitals or having orgasms, but also taking care of the other aspects of your sexuality—sexual pleasure and sexual satisfaction.

According to the World Association for Sexual Health (WAS), sexual health is "a state of physical, emotional, mental and social wellbeing in relation to sexuality; it is not merely the absence of disease, dysfunction or infirmity. Sexual health requires a positive and respectful approach to sexuality and sexual relationships, as well as the possibility of having pleasurable and safe sexual experiences, free of coercion, discrimination, and violence."

Sexuality is the core of your own being; it is who you are, whereas sex is just what you do sexually. According to WAS, "sexuality encompasses sex, gender identities, and roles, sexual orientation, eroticism, pleasure, intimacy, and reproduction. Sexuality is experienced and expressed in thoughts, fantasies, desires, beliefs, attitudes, values, behaviors, practices, roles, and relationships." Therefore, sexuality is an umbrella term for everything related to your sexual being, that is why it is the core of who you are. Remember, we are all sexual beings from before birth to death. Our sexuality is within us! Again, sex—sexual acts—is a part of sexuality, so sexuality is not based on sexual activities alone. It has much more to do with your mindset about sex, which we've talked about previously.

Now, what about your sexual rights? Sexual rights are part of Human Rights. To be sexually healthy, first and foremost, your sexual rights must be respected as well as your Human Rights. Most people do not realize that WAS has created a set of universal Sexual Rights to protect us, which can be found on their website: worldsexology.org. Once you know your sexual rights are being met, you can explore your sexuality in accordance with sexual health. If you understand these three things: your sexuality, sexual health, and your sexual rights, then you are free to experience sexual pleasure in your consensual relationships.

In 2019, the 24th World Association for Sexual Health (WAS) Congress was held in Mexico City. The declaration on Sexual Pleasure—found in Chapter 5—was the conclusion of this magnificent congress. The main theme and emphasis of the WAS Congress was the recognition of sexual pleasure as an essential element for our well-being. It was asserted that sexual pleasure is a central part of our existence and our sexual health, keeping in mind the necessity of consent and respect for all people.

Now, it is also important to be aware of the differences between healthy sex and unhealthy sex and distinguish them, for your sexual health, critical to your sexual happiness. Notice that healthy sex includes important elements, and one of them is sexual pleasure.

Healthy Sex

As I said before, healthy sex includes four important elements and these elements must always be present in any healthy sexual encounter, activity, or interaction of any kind. These four elements are: consent, responsibility, safety, and pleasure. So, healthy sex is ALWAYS:

Consensual
Responsible
Safe
Pleasurable

- ► Consensual: This means mutual agreement. ALL participants must agree on and consent to whatever you decide to do sexually. It is highly recommended that you be clear and aware of this before engaging in sexual activities or sex; that means, no alcohol or drugs involved that may alter judgment. Boundaries and limits must be clear as well.
- ► Responsible: This means being held accountable and being trustworthy, dependable, and well-informed, so your partner or partners involved can trust you, and everyone involved can assume the consequences of their actions.
- ► Safe: Sexual activities are all reliable, credible, and as risk free as possible. All participants are safe from harm and protected from STDs and/or unwanted pregnancy.
- ► Pleasurable: All participants are sexually free, expressing themselves in a pleasant, enjoyable, agreeable, delectable, and heartwarming way. There is no coercion, manipulation, obligation, exploitation, or infliction of emotional distress involved. People involved must feel respected and appreciated. Appreciation doesn't mean love; that is, feelings of love aren't a requisite for healthy sex, but respect, consent, and care for others are. Feeling good, comfortable, secure, relaxed, content, and happy is crucial to experience pleasure—that's the idea.

Sexual Dysfunctions, Problems, and Failures

Sexual dysfunctions, contrary to sexual failures, are persistent and recurrent—in every or almost every sexual activity, over a period of 6 months or more—difficulties when wanting to respond to a desired stimulus. Many times, individuals—men and women—may experience a sexual failure for any reason—we are humans—and they think they have got a problem, when in fact, they just were tired or something else. Failures are normal and happen to anyone.

But what happens when you or your partner are sick or don't take proper care of yourselves? What if you have a positive sexual mindset, but your body is not functioning as your mind would like it to? If you are experiencing a health problem, the sexual dysfunction can be a symptom of an underlying disease—medical conditions such as diabetes, heart and vascular disease, neurological disorders, etc.—not a sexual problem per se. The causes for sexual dysfunctions are not due to an underlying disease; they are real sexual problems and difficulties of a purely sexual nature—mental, physically, and/or relationship factors.

Sexual failures are momentary occasions where your genitals don't respond as expected during a certain moment, usually due to emotions such as anxiety, or because of temporary reactions from being tired, as I mentioned before. For instance, one of the most common psychological causes of erectile failures is "performance anxiety," as sex researchers Master & Johnson call it. This describes the spiral of self-doubt and anxiety you experience when you worry too much about your erections and sexual performance as a male. On the other hand, sexual dysfunctions are permanent situations that significantly affect you and your relationship. Something is not working! As explained by Helen Kaplan, MD, PhD, Clinical Professor of Psychiatry at the New York Hospital-Cornell Medical Center, "when these responses or any of their component phases are impaired, sexual dysfunction results."

A persistent and recurrent sexual problem that it is not being addressed, may mean that you are not quite sexually healthy. Where is your sexual health, then? Thus, you are not quite healthy in general. Your overall health is affected, even if you are eating properly, exercising, and sleeping well. Understanding sexuality, sexual rights, and sexual health includes how to overcome and face sexual problems the best you can, to free your sexual self positively and experience sexual pleasure. Find professional help if you are experiencing a sexual difficulty that has been persistent and recurrent over the past 6 months.

Life is rarely as easy as pie. It's not that simple, is it? We, as humans, usually complicate things, or things get complicated for us. We all want to be as healthy as possible, as well as productive, happy, and functional, but sometimes we do very little to accomplish that, either because we don't know what to do, we don't have enough information, or we don't fight enough to do whatever it takes to improve our conditions. So, being completely healthy, being in a fulfilling, committed relationship, and being very happy are not possible without effort; every aspect of yourselves should be worked on daily, with effort and energy!

Complications, failures, and problems may occur along the way—this is normal for all of us at some point of our lives—making things even more difficult, but not impossible! Happiness and pleasure must come from the inside out regardless of the outside circumstances. Be happy and have pleasure in your own unique way!

Think about Sarah and Frank, Case #2—their sexual mindset was good. They believed sex is positive and healthy. They had desires, fantasies, and open minds about sexuality. In general, they truly wanted to have a fulfilling sex life but couldn't. Sarah and Frank both had very poor health and did not take care of themselves properly. They both had unhealthy lifestyles, so their overall physical well-being was poor.

Therefore, they had neither the energy nor the enthusiasm to engage in sexual activities, even when they wanted to. When Sarah and Frank occasionally did it, their bodies could not function as they wished—due to their poor bodily conditions—leading to sexual problems.

Common Sexual Problems

Some people think that they are healthy even when experiencing a sexual problem. Nothing is further from the truth! If you have developed a sex problem, you will most likely avoid or stop having sex, missing the many great benefits of sex for your health, overall wellbeing, and your relationship. Therefore, you must overcome any impediment for enjoying your sexuality, and be able to *make love 365 times a year!*

There are many kinds of sexual problems; the most common is Low or Lack of Sexual Desire. Sexual problems have been divided into three main groups:

1. Desire problems—a lack of sexual desire or interest in sexual activities.
2. Arousal problems—the inability to be aroused during sexual activities you want.
3. Orgasm problems—no control over ejaculation. Absence of orgasm—called Pre-orgasmic.

1. Desire problems: Desire is a mental state. A desire problem happens when there is no motivation for sexual activities; you don't want sex, period. It is very common, and I often hear, especially from women, about the concern of not wanting to be sexually involved with their partner, or not wanting their partners—which does not necessarily mean that desire to be sexual has gone. Desire is curiosity and the willingness to explore sexually. It is not about hormones or age; it is about your mental state. Low desire is not a physical state—it is a lack of interest to explore, to feel, and to "go there."

In many cases, sexual desire is still present in a person's life, either spontaneously (comes naturally) or induced (it's provoked), but its manifestation is avoided, hidden, or neglected due to relationship conflicts, personal issues, false beliefs, repressed anger, or resentment. Therefore, it is to me, the most delicate problem to evaluate, since the concept is wrongly used to describe a person that just doesn't want to have sex anymore with a specific partner.

It is as Dr. Robert Birch, PhD, director of the Arlington Center for Marital and Sexual Concerns, says, "your lack of desire is not an illness, it's an eloquent expression of your feelings." Therefore, in my view, sexual problems are often expressions of relationship dissatisfaction, personal conflicts, negative conditioned responses, and/or negative feelings, which will be explored in the following chapter.

Problems start when one of you doesn't have a desire for sexual activities. Birch affirms that "it's only when there's a discrepancy in the desire that there's a problem." If you and your partner are happy and satisfied with the frequency you have sex, without forcing each other, then any frequency is fine, as long as both of you are happy. However, according to Braverman, the average healthy level of sexual frequency is three times per week. It is the sexual dose recommended by several sexologists, including me.

Sexual desire plays an important role in sexual frequency. I think it is highly important to deeply evaluate a lack of desire, by first distinguishing between: 1. Wanting to have sex but not having sexual interest or desire at all—wanting to want—and 2. Not wanting to have sex with a specific partner but having interest or the sexual desire. In that case, the problem becomes a *relationship problem* rather than a sexual problem, which should be faced as soon as possible for lasting sexual enjoyment.

Think about desire this way: you need strong sexual desire for great sex, but do you need strong sexual desire to make love and feel connected? If you deeply love your partner, why do you have to be "horny" or depend on your genitals to connect physically? If you want to make love and connect, then the desire to be close and connected should be stronger than the desire for just sex and orgasms. The desire to feel and explore your partner, the curiosity, and the interest to be together should always be present to *make love 365 times a year.*

Brazilian sexologist and psychologist Eliany Mariussi, author of *Na Cama Com a Sexologa,* suggested: "It seems men have more sexual desire than women—which we agree is not true—because culturally women were led not to like sex, not to think about it, not to talk about it, and mainly not to live their own sexuality, behaviors that have been reproduced until today." In fact, men and women have the same sexual needs and both experience fluctuations in sexual desire. It is a false belief that men are ready for sex 24/7. Men, as well as women, are affected by emotional and cultural stigmas, as well as context (environmental factors) such as work, relationship conflicts, children, and stress, that negatively impact their sexual desire—interest for sex. As a result, many men and women experience a decrease in energy as well due to hormonal imbalance and other organic factors, leading to wanting but not having the energy to act.

Thinking of your body as a car, a problem with desire would mean that you don't want to get in the car at all. You'd rather stay at home and not drive, period. Please, be aware of the difference between wanting to desire versus desiring but not wanting to desire. In any case, if your goal is to *make love 365 times a year,* the desire—the interest—to be with your partner and feel them is important.

2. Arousal problems: This is a physical state where your body is not physically responding for organic and/or psychological reasons. You want to have sex; you have the desire to have sex but can't get started.

For men the issue is usually the inability to have or maintain a firm enough erection to engage in sexual intercourse, known as Erectile Dysfunction (ED).

For women, it is usually a lack of excitement, causing sexual pain. The use of lubricant helps in great deal when there is desire but not enough lubrication, which is perfectly fine. Remember that in most cases, especially among women, there is no concordance between how you feel and your body's response, such as lubrication. This means that a woman can be mentally aroused and not lubricated, and vice versa. Therefore, the physical response should never be more important than the *mental desire* of what a person—woman or man—wants.

Erectile Dysfunction (ED) probably gets the most attention of all the sexual problems because it is the one with more publicity. The penis is not responding to proper sexual stimuli, causing severe mental distress and relationship problems. Arousal problems would be like getting into the car and not being able to crank it or having the battery die. Therefore, taking proper care of your health is essential for optimal sexual functioning, for both men and women.

3. Orgasm problems: This is a mental and physical state where your body responds in an unwanted way, or too fast, too slow, or not at all. An orgasm problem would be the car going too fast, too slow, or never reaching a destination.

   ► A too fast response is called Rapid Ejaculation (RE), where the plateau stage is too short or non-existent. Usually men have no control over their ejaculation.
   ► A too slow response is called Delayed Ejaculation, where men have a hard time ejaculating or orgasming.
   ► A total lack of response is called Pre-Orgasmic: an inability to experience orgasm in any wanted sexual encounter, including masturbation. This can happen to men, but mostly happens to women.

Rapid Ejaculation (RE) is, to me, the most easy and fun problem to treat—when it isn't a symptom of an underlying disease. It is about training rather than treatment. It is a sexual problem—not an illness—where there is no control or awareness over the ejaculatory process, affecting both, the individual and his partner. According to my experience, a couple working together on RE, not only overcome the problem but also gain an immense sexual intimacy, better knowledge of each other, and a stronger connection.

On the other hand, Delayed Ejaculation is less common, and it can be due to an organic problem. However, according to my experience, it is a problem mostly related to negative thoughts, anxiety, and/or lack of proper sexual stimulation, including poor sexual fantasies.

For men who have difficulty ejaculating, I recommend focusing on feelings and sensations, having longer periods of exciting foreplay before intercourse, increasing sexual fantasies, and training yourself to experience orgasm without ejaculating; that is, to learn to separate orgasm from ejaculation in order to be able to enjoy multiple orgasms. Not too bad when *making love 365 times a year...*

Conditioned Negative Sexual Responses

As I mentioned before, we, human, complicate things! One perfect example of complicating things is the formation of conditioned negative sexual responses that contribute to sexual problems. We have conditioned responses to certain stimuli, responses that are created in our childhood and adolescence years.

For instance, when you go from a natural response—a normal, spontaneous response—to a conditioned negative one after experiencing negative feelings. The initial response is called a spontaneous response. This is the natural response your body gives if it has no prior experience with the stimuli. Once you have associated that stimuli with the experience, be it positive or negative, you will create a conditioned response to that stimuli. This is true for sexually conditioned responses as well.

Therefore, a conditioned response is an alteration in response, a new modified response you have created AFTER learning to associate a certain experience with certain stimuli—usually a bad experience. A typical example can be the association of food with pleasure or disgust. For instance, the association of apple pie's smell with mouthwatering, hunger, or memories of your grandmother's home. But say you got sick off apple pie, unconsciously creating a bad memory and forming a new response to apple pie—now a conditioned response: you may feel ill instead of delighted when smelling apple pies.

The same is true for sexually conditioned responses. If you begin to associate sex and sexual practices with something negative due to previous negative experiences, feelings, or beliefs, you probably aren't having a natural sexual response to sexual stimuli. You are instead having a negative conditioned response to any sexual activity, unconsciously creating your new normal response, leading to loads of sexual problems.

Sexual Responses

What, then, is a natural reaction to a sexual stimulus? It is when a flaccid penis transforms into an erect phallus, or a dry vaginal space becomes a wet, engorged space when it is properly stimulated. Initial sexual reactions build off one another, leading to sexual activities. Sex doesn't just happen; some steps are needed—such as desire and arousal—before engaging in sexual acts. But, if you have negative conditioned sexual response, probably you will stop at some point to avoid the negative sensations. I will talk about these steps or phases involved in the circle of sexual response later in Chapter 7.

Sexual problems are all about your body's sexual responses, about not being able to fully sexually react/respond to a specific pleasant sexual stimulus. When thinking of your body as the vehicle, remember that you want a vehicle that works properly. Your ability to respond shows that your body is functioning properly.

Usually, we begin the sexual "playing" having the desire—curiosity—to "go there." Then we must turn on the "vehicle," your body, just as we would with a car. You can't go anywhere with the car off! Once on, you will have more desire and will want more. In this way you will "drive" your body, aroused and wanting, to the direction that you most want, and eventually, you will "get there," to your destination in a satisfactory and pleasurable way. This is what I mean by proper functioning.

Sometimes when having a poor sexual response—like no feeling aroused or the inability to maintain an erection—you might panic and think you have a sexual problem. But again, if you don't know your body, how can you assume you have a problem? By believing so, you may then create a real problem in your mind as if it were an absolute fact, forming a toxic sex habit that will be reinforced next time it happens.

Please, don't think of the problems as right or wrong or good or bad; think about whether your body is working the way you want. And if not, why?

Be Sexually Healthy and Enjoy Your Sexuality

Ejaculation and orgasms are important, and they should not be taken for granted. For instance, studies have shown that regular ejaculation in men reduces the chances of developing prostate cancer. An Australian study showed that men who ejaculated 21 times a month were less likely to develop cancer. Similarly, other researches have shown that having frequent sex reduces the risk of prostate and breast cancer as well and support your immune system.

Studies have found that about 10% of women are Pre-Orgasmic; that is, they have never experienced an orgasm in their lives. A study in the University of Pittsburgh found that 63 percent of women who said they were happily married had trouble reaching orgasm or becoming aroused. Orgasms are important, but not the essential part or the purpose of lovemaking. If a negative or problematic sexual responses have become "normal" for you—your conditioned sexual responses—they are unintentional and unconscious, so you may not be aware that you really have a problem to overcome; you believe it is "normal." Therefore, sexual problems may become okay for you, normal and habitual, making you comfortable with them.

If this is the case for you, I recommend you do something for your sexual health, since this situation is not positive at all! Having sexual problems is unhealthy. They bring sexual apathy, frustration, and disconnection from your partner, if you have one, as well as from your own sexual self. If you are in a relationship, and both of you as a couple are experiencing sexual problems, one of the main contributing factors is often the relationship itself. Think about your car again—your partner is the one in the car with you. If you don't want him/her in the car with you, then you are not going anywhere, or it will be a long rough ride! You will not be making love, but war!

If you're indifferent or angry at your partner, you won't be sexually intimate. Many couples see only the sexual problem they have, rather than their relationship as the source of the problem. Then, they—usually the guy—want to "fix" the partner, so that they become "more sexual." This is a disaster! In this case, the sexual problem is only a symptom. If it is treated as a problem, the total process will fail, leading to more frustration or even a breakup.

Researcher and professor of psychiatry and behavioral neuroscience, Dr. Richard Balon, MD, has done studies to show the cost of sexual dysfunctions. According to Balon, there is not just the financial burden that comes with illness, but the loss of quality of life as well. We are talking about QUALITY of life, not just the years in your life. Sexual problems can lead to poor quality of life, loss of relationships, an increase in anxiety and/or depression, and potential embarrassment, affecting personal confidence and self-esteem.

For instance, men suffering from RE and/or ED report all sorts of issues with depression and anxiety that lead to lower satisfaction with life, and surprisingly, their partners report the same! Women are just as affected psychologically by their male's partners sexual dysfunctions. Moreover, women are most likely to experience low desire. According to Balon, "women suffering from this dysfunction report everything, from anxiety and depression to difficulty conceiving."

We all want to not only live longer but live longer and better, right?

Sex is an essential component of physical and mental well-being. Many people don't even refer to their sexual health. They think only about their genitals—especially men, who tend to be penis-oriented, looking for sexual release. But sexual health is so much more than this. You are and will always be a sexual being—from the time you are born, even before you are born, until you die. Even if you aren't in a relationship, sexuality and your sexual health are still important. It is important regardless of your age, race, gender, or whether you're in a relationship. Only when you are taking care of your sexuality as well as your overall health can you say you are truly healthy. If you want a full quality of life, you should have a fulfilling sex life.

Benefits of a Healthy Sex Life

Recent studies show the multiple benefits that an active sex life brings to health. Dr. Shelley, PhD, explains in *Anti-Aging & Health Benefits of Sex* the physical, emotional, anti-aging, and spiritual benefits of sex. As Shelley says, "sex can help the individual stay young, and keep relationships vibrant and alive…frequent sex and sexual activity can help reduce the effects of aging and keep-you-healthier."

Research at North Carolina State University suggests that there could be an important link between the act of fellatio—oral sex performed on male—and breast cancer. The researchers found that those who performed the act of fellatio regularly, one to two times a week, had a lower occurrence of breast cancer than those who did not. One of the researchers, Dr. Helena Shifteer, concluded that "only with regular occurrence will your chances be reduced, so I encourage all women out there to make fellatio an important part of their daily routine. Since the emergence of the research, I try to fellate at least once every other night to reduce my chances."

It has been shown that there are many benefits of semen for humans. Semen is pure and very healthy—when a man eats well and doesn't smoke. Semen is a protein fluid rich in potassium, iron, calcium, lecithin, enzymes, minerals, vitamins—including vitamin E—phosphorus, proteins, testosterone, and other hormones and essentials. It has been scientifically proven to have anxiolytics (anti-anxiety) and anti-cancer effects, as a researcher has shown. It's not bad at all! It is great for everything!

Furthermore, Levin's 2003 research found that vaginal intercourse helps maintain vaginal and pelvic function. There were also indications that semen in the vagina helps maintain vaginal oxygenation and blood flow. As Shelley wrote, "ejaculation may actually keep the vagina healthy. Increased sexual activity can help keep you healthy 'down there'." Hence, the consumption of semen should be considered, as Shifteer recommends, by swallowing it through fellatio, by absorbing it through the vaginal walls right after intercourse—without a condom—or in food/drinks as suggested by Paul "Fotie" Photenhauer in his book *Semenology.*

I have had clients over 80 years old who come to me looking for ways to still be sexually active and healthy, to keep themselves in the "game of love," no matter what! They are fighting for an excellent quality of life and continuing to make love or have sex. Their desire to improve themselves, their sex life, and their relationships is beautiful and outstanding to me. From them, I have learned to never give up, even for a second, to stay sexually active, to enjoy more, and to live longer and happier!

Improve the quality of your love life through a healthy lifestyle, as I mentioned before. Not everything can be money, politics, work, business—even family. More important than all of that should be your love life, your health, and your happiness. As Braverman suggests, "by keeping an active sex life, you'll feel more vibrant, smarter, more loving, and enjoy better sleep. You'll also have a greater incentive to be healthier, fitter, and thinner."

We can conclude here that being healthy helps you to have more and better sex, and having frequent sex makes you healthier. It is a fantastic circuit that feeds itself: health helps you to have good sex, and good sex helps you to stay healthy. So, health promotes sex and sex promotes health.

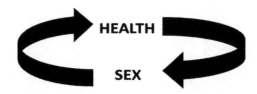

Health leads to sex and sex leads to health.

See some of the many benefits of having HEALTHY SEX:

- ▶ Facilitates the skin's ability to produce vitamin D
- ▶ Helps the brain function quicker and better
- ▶ Reduces anxiety and depression
- ▶ Helps with better sleep
- ▶ Decreases the risk of breast cancer and prostate cancer
- ▶ Lessens the frequency of hot flashes in menopause
- ▶ Raises estradiol levels and stimulates blood flow
- ▶ Raises oxytocin and endorphins and lower cortisol, thus lowering stress
- ▶ Leads to a better relationship
- ▶ Smooths the skin, calm the mind, relieve stress and restore a sense of humor
- ▶ Improves self-esteem
- ▶ Keeps motivation to stay sexy and attractive

Sex, then, is wealth! Right? It is something excellent for all of us. Your body has an impact on your whole life; it is your unique singular vehicle to drive for your entire life! So, you should keep your unique vehicle in good condition, the best you can, for a functional and pleasurable love life to *make love 365 times a year.*

Yale sociologist and professor of sociology at the University of Washington, Pepper Schwartz, PhD, and et al, suggest in *The Normal Bar,* that "we somehow find the discipline to exercise, dress well, eat right, and keep our energy high. We try to look attractive…but we let other priorities take over…no more time and effort into looking great for our partners." Don't allow that to happen to you; prioritize your health and love life, no matter what!

Start today; love yourself, have fun, and *make love 365 times a year!* It's never too late.

—Dr. Heinz

Part V: 7 Suggestions & Recommended Sources

7 Simple Suggestions for a Healthy You

1. Start forming healthy love habits. For example, the first thing to do every morning is to be grateful for your life and your unique body. Secondly, deeply kiss and hug your partner good morning—a love habit that I call "Pretzel Time." This strengthens your connection every day. I do these things, even if I slept through the alarm or know I have a busy day. Third, drink water. Try to keep a large water bottle close to you. Next, have a healthy breakfast. There is a correlation between brain health and a good, healthy breakfast. Also, five minutes of stretching is good to get your blood flowing and get ready for the day.

2. Have morning sex! Have morning sex as part of your routine, as a love habit! Morning sex improves the functioning of your organs, multiplies and strengthens antibodies, improves circulation and lowers blood pressure—and thus, the risk of heart disease decreases. Oxytocin release is guaranteed, which will keep you connected through the day. What a way to start your day!!

3. Work step-by-step on building a healthy lifestyle and a strong self-esteem in order to feel great. Self-esteem is one of my favorite topics in my practice. There are many pillars to self-esteem, and the first one is self-knowledge! Start by knowing yourself—the real you—and accepting the way you are. This applies to knowing your sexual self. Masturbation is essential to know your true self and start building good self-esteem. But please, do it without using porn; use only your imagination.

4. You are responsible for your sexual health…be careful of what you feed your body, mind, and spirit. Remember that you are a sexual being. Sexuality is part of who you are. Don't waste precious time holding back your sexual desires. Give your best. Inspire others, especially your partner, to be sexually responsible, active, and safe. Practice healthy sex—always. Let your meaningful sexual wisdom guide you. Put your heart in your sexual path…

5. Have FREQUENT SEX to protect your prostate—or your partner's prostate—and your overall well-being! Frequent ejaculations are important and healthy. The prostate gland secretes most of the fluid you ejaculate. If you don't ejaculate, the fluid stays in the gland, which tends to swell, causing lots of problems. Regular ejaculation will wash those fluids out and ensure the well-being of your prostate until old age. Also, frequent sexual activity reduces stress, the chances of cancer, and other conditions, for both men and women.

6. Have plenty of orgasms per week; I recommend three orgasms per week. Remember, orgasms benefit the circulatory, neural, muscular, articular, and hormonal systems as well as the Genito-urinary system. Sexual health enriches the quality of our lives! Practice solo sex regularly, without compulsion, to know and appreciate your sexuality, as I recommended before—without the use of porn. Your orgasms are your responsibility, not your partner's!

7. There are no magic pills for good sex, for being healthy, or for staying sexy. But the truth is, you and only you have the power to eat well and have a great sex life. The real aphrodisiacs are good foods full of nutrients that allow optimal sexual performance—and, of course, a sexy partner! Once you've begun eating healthy, exercising, and sleeping well, everything else will follow. Keep going and remember that it's never too late, or too early for a better love life!

Recommended Sources for Sex Secret #2

Neuroloveology: The Power to Mindful Love & Sex by Ava Cadell, Ph.D.

10 Signs you Know What Matters Article by Steven C. Hayes, Ph.D.

Sex Matters by Louanne Cole Weston, Ph.D.

Younger (Thinner) You Diet by Dr. Eric R. Braverman, MD.

Simple Sexy Food: 101 Tasty Aphrodisiac Recipes and Sensual Tips to Stir Your Libido and Feed Your Love by Linda De Villers, Ph.D.

Change your Brain chance your Life by Dr. Daniel Amen

Come As You Are: The Surprising New Science That Will Transform Your Sex Life by Emily Nagoski, Ph.D.

Elite Minds by Dr. Stan Beecham

The Practical Encyclopedia of Sex and Heath by Stefan Bechtel

The Normal Bar: The Surprising Secrets of Happy Couples and What They Reveal About Creating a New Normal in Your Relationship by Pepper Schwartz, Ph.D., et al

Anti-Aging & Health Benefits of Sex by Dr. Shelley, Ph.D.

Semenology by Paul "Fotie" Photenhauer

The Longevity Paradox: How to Die Young at a Ripe Old Age by Dr. Steven R. Gundry, MD.

What The Health by Kip Andersen and Keegan Kuhn

Fellatio May Significantly Decrease the Risk of Breast Cancer in Women by Dr. Helena Shifteer et all. A study by North Carolina State University

World Association for Sexual Health (WAS). Website: http://www.worldsexo logy.org/

Na Cama Com a Sexologa: Problemas Sexuais Enfrentados Pelos Casais by Eliany Mariussi (Portuguese)

SEX SECRET 3

CHAPTER 3

Loving Feelings

>——————————————>

The supreme happiness of life is the conviction that we are loved.
—Victor Hugo

Sex is always about emotions. Good sex is about free
emotions, bad sex is about blocked emotions.
—Deepak Chopra

Part I: Feelings Toward Your Partner

The feelings you have for each other have a tremendous impact on your sex life. You cannot make love with resentment and repressed feelings in your heart. The most widespread problem among couples today that drastically interferes in their sex life is, according to my professional experience, resentment.

Resentment is hard feelings that one partner holds against the other, and this can damage a relationship. Feelings of anger, fear, doubt, disgust, hurt, or hatred are very destructive, and they can kill your love life completely. Resentment, to me, is the "relationship cancer," and according to my professional experience, it is the number one problem couples face today, which leads to disconnection, sexual dissatisfaction, breakups, infidelity, and even divorce.

I have encountered throughout my entire career as a counselor that no matter the culture, age, race, economic and intellectual status, or education of my clients, undealt-with resentment is your sex life's worse enemy, which will prevent you from making love. Instead, good and positive feelings and thoughts are your best friend, fundamental for sustaining a healthy sex life. This chapter, then, is the heart of this book, and of my work...

Let's see what happened to John and Alexa, Case #3.

Case #3: John & Alexa

John, age 43, and Alexa, age 38, have been married for seven years and knew each other for six before that. Together they have a three-year-old son. Their lifestyle includes healthy eating, dogs, steady jobs, and a nice house.

Quickly I realized they both have good and positive sexual mindsets (Sex Secret #1). And a great healthy lifestyle (Sex Secret #2).

John and Alexa used to have a very active sex life—the key phrase is "USED to have." Both believed that sex is helpful for a healthy life and were open about their own sexuality. But their sex life has fallen by the wayside. There were no obvious answers to their problem, as they were both healthy, fit, going to the gym, eating well, etc. They had an active life and healthy lifestyles, they cared for each other, and they had college degrees and successful careers.

John immediately told me why they came to see me.

"I want to improve our sex life; I want it to be as before."

Alexa agreed. "We've been having less and less sex over time."

I ask about their son.

"It isn't because of him," Alexa answered confidently.

"Well...I get irritated when Alexa pushes me away," John continued. "I want the same sex that we've always had. I still love her and want her. I don't know what happened..."

"Alexa just shrugs it off," John continued.

Then Alexa added, "right now, I don't feel like it. I don't have any drive to engage in sex. I've always been sexual, but now I don't want any more; I'm pissed off."

She seems to think for a second.

"We don't have time together. We don't!"

I could see John getting visibly irritated beside her.

"She has no clue what's going on," he accused.

Since nothing seemed to be coming to light, I asked to talk to them individually. John didn't say anything clarifying, except that he didn't know what happened. Alexa told me a different story.

I started by asking if she still wanted to be sexually with him, "the desire to desire him, the want to want..."

"Yes!" she answered.

To make sure, and to pinpoint exactly what was happening in our individual session, I asked Alexa about her sexuality. She was still masturbating and had sexual fantasies. She simply did not want to share these times with her husband anymore. Objectively, she still wanted him and was still attracted to him, but I found out that her resentment prevented her from being sexually intimate with him.

So, the problem was not low desire due to unhealthy conditions, nor her beliefs about sex, but her feelings toward her husband. Then, I started asking about the past.

"When I was pregnant, he wasn't a help...wasn't emotionally present for me," she finally tells me. "He wasn't a total jerk either; he didn't call me names or anything like that, or say I disgusted him, but he wasn't helpful. He didn't take care of me like I thought he would; he really was absent, in his own world."

Alexa continued to tell me that his disinterest and apathy during her pregnancy had caused her to resent him for years. Apparently, they never talked about it.

"And once the baby was here, he became very detached. Suddenly, he started playing tennis or was always at work. The baby was MY problem, not his. He just was our provider."

Crying as she remembered this, she got to the root of the problem.

"I suffered alone with the baby, our baby..."

With an emotionally unavailable, and sometimes physically absent partner, people suffer, as in the case of Alexa. She felt overwhelmed and abandoned by her partner–her husband John. She had never talked about this; instead, time passed without resolution. That created an invisible wall, called resentment, which she was unable to scale.

John didn't understand what was happening, so he started to resent his wife as well, making them seem more detached from one another. This caused Alexa to become angrier, which made him more frustrated. They had created a vicious cycle of negative feelings without realizing it. Now that John was traveling more for work, they were spending even more time apart, which lead to their disconnection.

This also led them to not having sex at all!

Alexa still loved him but did not want to be sexually intimate with her husband because of her hard feelings toward him. I told her that it was their resentment that was standing in the way of their love life. Once she had hidden these feelings away, they had begun to fester. It's like if you're holding a "rotten fish." The WORST thing you can do is shove that fish in a drawer and throw away the key. The smell and the fish will only get worse. When you finally open the drawer, the problem seems insurmountable.

Couples often become non-sexual because of resentment. I have learned from my clients always to make sure there are no hidden negative feelings between them. Frequently this can take multiple sessions, separately, or more often, together. Sometimes they both have resentment, but usually one of them doesn't even know that "there's a fish in the drawer!"

Studies show a strong correlation between a fulfilling relationship and sexual satisfaction. Negative feelings about your relationship and/or your partner are detrimental for your sexual fulfillment. Therefore, your feelings toward your partner are, in my opinion, the most crucial and important Sex Secret of all! It is very difficult, if not impossible, to *make love 365 times a year* while holding resentment and negative feelings toward each other. You and your partner—both of you—must clean them up before making love. To make love, you need "clean" LOVE!

By now, you should have checked your sexual mindset (Sex Secret #1) and your health and physical condition (Sex Secret #2).

In this chapter, Chapter 3, your feelings towards your partner will be examined, as well as the emotions affecting those feelings. We will explore what sex really is, what lovemaking is, the feeling of romantic love, and the importance of trusting your partner.

So, let's start with these questions:

▶ How do you feel about and around your partner?
▶ Do you feel totally comfortable, relaxed, truthful, and secure when you are together?
▶ What do you think about your partner when you are together? When you are apart?
▶ Are you holding resentment? Unsolved issues?
▶ Does your partner/spouse feel the same way you feel?
▶ How does your partner feel about you? Please, don't guess, ASK! It is very important to know, so don't be afraid to talk about your feelings.

Sex Secret #3 is all about loving feelings you should have for your partner, and how to become emotionally healthy in order to *make love 365 times a year!* You might have dislikes toward other people, your family members, or even the entire world, but it is with your partner with whom you are supposed to make love. Right?

Negative feelings block feelings of love…

When I ask for feelings, the typical answer I get is usually the instinctual reaction: "Of course I love my partner!" But this answer is expected. If someone is at my practice trying to fix their sex life, then it's evident, to me, that they still have some good feelings—they are trying to do something about it. If the feelings of love were completely gone, they wouldn't be coming to see me; they would be finding a divorce lawyer!

Case #3 illustrates these typical problems couples face that prevent them from having a healthy sex life. I have had the privilege of helping thousands of couples like John and Alexa to overcome resentments, throughout my years of practice, resulting in the total restoration of their intimacy, sex life, and passion.

Let's look at Alexa's and John's Lovemaking Wheels. Please observe how low they both scored on Loving Feelings:

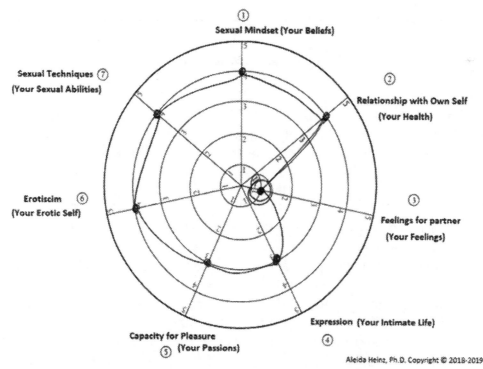

Aleida Heinz, Ph.D. Copyright © 2018-2019

Alexa's Lovemaking Wheel. Wheel #5

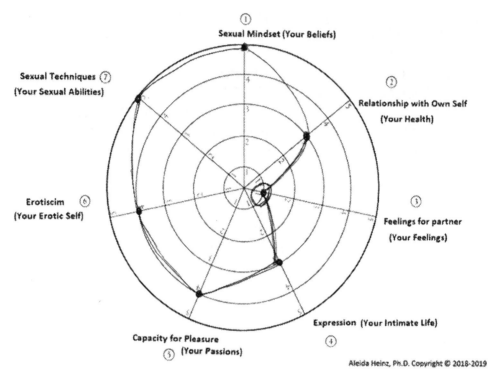

Sexual Mindset (Your Beliefs)

Sexual Techniques (7)
(Your Sexual Abilities)

Relationship with Own Self
(Your Health)

Erotiscim (6)
(Your Erotic Self)

Feelings for partner
(Your Feelings)

Expression (Your Intimate Life)

Capacity for Pleasure
(Your Passions)

Aleida Heinz, Ph.D. Copyright © 2018-2019

John's Lovemaking Wheel. Wheel #6

I hope the readings of this chapter will help you explore your feelings and keep them positive, with no resentment, in order to *make love 365 times a year*, as John and Alexa did after working hard on "emptying the emotional talk."

Resentment

Always keep in mind that resentment is hard feelings toward someone. Even if you wish to make love, you can't because of these negative feelings or "rotten fish" between you and your partner won't allow that. This happens to both men and women, but in my experience, women hold onto resentment most often. Usually, men tend to forget the hard feelings, especially when they want to have sex, but women keep and hold on to them. Feelings of hatred and resentment only bring stress and unpleasantness, which in turn bring doubt, distrust, insecurity, and uneasiness, preventing people from openness and closeness.

Who wants to make love while feeling bad? Usually, negativity pushes people away, and your partner is not an exception!

Likewise, purely positive feelings bring easiness, trust, desire, and closeness, so that people can be open to love and make love. Isn't it what you want? If so, then work on your resentment first!

If you do not make the effort to get over your negative feelings, letting these experiences go unresolved and the feelings unventilated could cause an invisible wall between both of you, and eventually desire will die and resentment will grow, disconnecting you on many levels. As VS Glen, one of the writers for Talk About Marriage says, "don't let things fall to the wayside or they may sow the seeds of resentment, and that is a surefire way to kill a marriage." Remember Dr. Birch from Chapter 2: "Your lack of desire is not an illness, it's an eloquent expression of your *feelings.*" Understand, then, that the non-expression of your negative feelings and resentment affects your sex life.

Harsh feelings could have been created from diverse sources or experiences throughout your relationship, like in the case of John and Alexa. The most common difficult experience couples face in a relationship, that tends to disconnect them, is pregnancy—especially if unwanted. Parenthood, infidelity—a major one—negativity, mental problems, financial problems, inaction, laziness or behavioral problems, substance abuse, and unwanted extended family, among others, are typical difficulties that many couples go through, creating hard feelings.

Prevent resentments by facing your problems immediately! It is the only effective way to "empty your emotional tank" or get rid of your "rotten fish." If not, in the worse-case scenario, outside people and/or activities become the solution to emotional loneliness to survive–for a while. The results? Emotional detachment, isolation, disconnection, and the emergence of a "roommate style" relationship. Lovemaking will no longer be possible, replaced instead with fucking each other occasionally, causing couples to end up in a sexless and unhealthy relationship. Remember our visual of the car. Your sexual mindset is your GPS and your body the vehicle. Now, your feelings for each other is the route your vehicle drives along. It is up to you where the route goes, but your feelings determine how clear and easy your road will be.

Your feelings should be as a "smooth German highway" where you can drive with no speed limit in total freedom, with the certainty that you're going to get to wherever you want to go. Or the opposite—your feelings can become like a "bumpy dirt road" where you will find many obstacles and problems preventing you from happily reaching your destination.

Let's examine your route. Is it in good shape? Do you and your partner have any hard feelings that haven't been resolved? Many times, couples put their uncomfortable feelings aside because they believe those feelings will disappear or get better over time. Not true! Many people don't talk about their negative feelings—instead, they talk about everything else to avoid conflict or being hurt. But silence is worse; it only brings more resentment and disconnection. By thinking you'll be okay by not talking, you are just making things worse; you will be creating a "bumpy road."

Again, hard feelings just grow worse and worse if you hide them; they get rotten and fester the longer they're hidden until they become resentment: "the dead fish in the drawer." This resentment will only go away if you face it. Understand that when you don't talk, your feelings only get worse, and these feelings are your route! You'll have no clue what is going on...

You'll need professional help to overcome strong anger, like in the case of being cheated on, because the pain produced is usually too much to handle alone. Unresolved anger gets hardened and becomes a stone between you and your partner. These stones may have now deepened and expanded, making the route to lovemaking impassable. Small slights also can grow into giant boulders. You'll need to remove any stones out of your route. It isn't easy, but the work is required for a smooth "German highway." Only then can you enjoy a fantastic trip to *making love 365 times a year*!

Let's smooth out the feelings toward each other (the road) to a fulfilling destination!

Please, avoid creating resentment at all costs if you want to make love! One of the behaviors that typically generate great resentment is infidelity, which is the leading cause of loss of trust. Trust and surrender are essential to lovemaking, and the reciprocity of love is as important as trust. But what happens when trust is broken in your relationship? How else can you surrender to your partner without trust?

Infidelity and Trust

In most cases, infidelity destroys relationships or forces them to change, for better or worse. Usually, I see infidelity as a symptom of underlying problems such as lack of emotional and/or sexual intimacy, loneliness, disconnection, resentment, etc.—although not necessarily. This situation may cause partners to deeply evaluate their relationship—in the best scenario. The outcome will depend on how the situation is perceived and whether emotions are handled properly.

What exactly is infidelity? How can infidelity impact your sex life? How do you overcome the suffering from infidelity? Is it possible? How long does it take to recover from it? Is it healthy to continue with the same unfaithful partner, or to have sex with them after infidelity has occurred? Does infidelity only affect couples in closed relationships? How do emotions and feelings change after an affair? These are important questions people ask me when being cheated on that you must consider, even before wondering whether it could happen to you—proactive prevention!

The basic definition of infidelity refers to the violation of trust and agreements made between partners which should not be confused by adultery. Some people see infidelity as identical as adultery. It is not! These two terms are associated, but they are not synonymous with one another. Adultery is more of a legal term that explicitly points out intercourse with someone else. Infidelity is simply breaking the agreements and the trust your partner has in you. The exact definition—or the line that can't be crossed—will vary from couple to couple. To determine what infidelity means for you, you must talk to your partner. This talk, though difficult, will lead to more trust.

Psychotherapist Esther Perel has made a great contribution to the understanding of infidelity. In *The State of Affairs: Rethinking Infidelity* she says, "an affair is an act of betrayal; it is the fact that the behavior is not within the couple's agreement. It is a 'violation of trust' that involves three fundamental elements: Secrecy, Sexual alchemy, and Emotional involvement."

Secrecy is the cornerstone of infidelity. It is the key element that turns a situation into infidelity. It is the secret that one partner hides that hurts the relationship the most and hurts the other partner as well. It is about creating a double life. According to most of my clients, it is the lies that hurt the most and are much worse than the unfaithful act itself. When cheating, you are concentrating so hard on those lies, and putting so much energy into not being discovered, that it will be hard to focus on your partner. Remember from Chapter 1 how important focus is! If you are hiding and lying it will be very difficult to connect.

Please, don't confuse secrecy with privacy, though. Secrecy deals with something your partner doesn't know about, whereas privacy deals with something they do know about, but you do not discuss—such as going to the bathroom. If, within your agreement, you agree that watching porn isn't infidelity, the fact that you give your partner privacy to watch it is not secrecy. You know about the porn; you are simply not a part of the proceedings.

Infidelity and the Internet

Researchers have found that 70% of men and 50% of women will be unfaithful at some point, which means that 80% of marriages will deal with one partner having an affair. The most likely places for these affairs to begin are the workplace and the Internet. According to recent research, two-thirds of married people are currently using the Internet for cybersex.

Some people think behaviors on the Internet can't be cheating because you aren't touching one another and are far apart. Pedro and I, authors of *The In-Factor Model How Internet Can Lead to Infidelity* found out that the Internet may lead to infidelity because intimacy and emotional connection are at play. In *The In-Factor Model*, we state that "infidelity is a strong sign that one partner is trying to escape emotionally." We interviewed couples in open and closed relationships who were dealing with infidelity. Around 40% of these couples had experienced fights to the point of divorce, and more than 50% saw no improvement in their sex life. They found it difficult to return to the relationship they had before infidelity occurred.

As Perel says, "transgression is the heart of human nature...the Internet has made it easy for people in committed relationships to transgress anytime and anywhere, usually just for simple curiosity which leads them to secrecy." Infidelity, to one person, can be flirting with someone on the Internet, kissing a stranger, or a backrub with an old friend, while others can see infidelity as nothing else but penetrative sex with someone outside the relationship.

To know exactly what infidelity is for you, talk about the explicit agreements that you and your partner have made. Consider, think, learn, and talk about the following factors:

- ▶ Attraction towards other people (those you know, as well as strangers).
- ▶ People you talk to or meet on Facebook, Instagram, or other Internet sites.
- ▶ People you talk with from your past, especially exes.
- ▶ Porn, cybersex, etc.
- ▶ Erotic massages, clubs, and any other places that provide sex and/or happy endings.

Then, you will know what your partner believes infidelity is, and where the line is drawn in your relationship. You aren't going in blind and just assuming that what you believe is "too far" is the same for your partner.

Overcoming Infidelity

Extreme emotions that go on too long can undermine your mental stability. Studies have found that when you are in a bad place and something triggers an emotional response—like infidelity—the subsequent emotions become highly intense. According to Perel "infinite reactions such as confusion, fear, pain, struggle, hurt, sadness, contradictions, anger, jealousy, shame, guilt, indignation, uncertainty, agony, and especially mistrust" are consequences of infidelity. So, be careful when triggering intense emotions; you never know how your partner will react.

If you or your partner have transgressed on the agreements you've made to one another, and decide you want to repair your relationship rather than end it, you will have to face the lies and suffering that have occurred. You both must work through all feelings of despair from infidelity before trying to make love again. Repair must occur. I agree with Perel that "repair is to re-pair." You need to start over with a different level of consciousness and awareness. Sexologist, clinical psychologist, sex therapist, and author of *Extraordinary Sex Now*, Sandra Scantling, PhD, advises that "the first ingredient for extraordinary sex is to put away all old hurts and anger...anger blocks intimacy. Just as each of us is responsible for our own pleasure, the same is true for our own hostility."

Putting away all hurt is essential to *make love 365 times a year.* And intimacy is the foundation to regaining trust again. I suggest you do these four things:

1. Put away the pain: Those hard and negative feelings. Give yourself room to heal. It takes time. Crying is not bad, it heals.
2. Get back the love and trust: You used to have love for your partner. Remember those days! Talking is the first step to this.
3. Find your identity and your relationships' identity again: Without being in denial, re-invent yourself. People sometimes confuse trusting their partner with blindness to their faults. This is denial. Face reality and learn to trust without turning a blind eye to errors.
4. Find professional help! Friends and family may want to help, they probably have good intentions, but they cannot be impartial in their

opinions. Don't allow your life, your health, and overall happiness to be ruined.

This topic is crucial. You must be sure you have gotten over the ugly ghost of infidelity to make love in the future. Don't put "this fish in the drawer" and expect it to go away—it will only stink worse the longer you ignore it. While cheating doesn't automatically mean divorce, it does mean the death of your lovemaking, which may lead to divorce if not addressed.

From my practice, I can tell you how difficult and exhausting it is to get trust and good feelings back after infidelity has happened. It is a lot of hard work for the couple to get over this issue. Therefore, think carefully before you transgress against your partner, because sooner or later the nefarious consequences will arise. It is like being pregnant; eventually, it will be noticed. I am not saying that cheating is evil, right, or wrong. But you must know that if you choose—because it is a choice—to go against the agreements you have made with your partner, then there will probably be a cascade of horrific emotions that will follow you afterwards, no matter what you do.

Preventing Infidelity

Prevention is always better than cure. Even if infidelity hasn't occurred in your relationship, it is a ghost that threatens all relationships, open or closed. It's important that you still talk about this idea with your partner before it is too late. What are your needs? Your partner's needs? Be aware that broken trust can destroy your sex life and probably your marriage too, so deal with it before it happens.

I have observed, analyzed, and concluded that infidelity comes from poor or non-connection, either emotional or sexual; lack of agreement; poor communication; bad handling of attractions and opportunities that arise, and lack of consequences. Being faithful is a decision, and to maintain this decision, you need to have willpower, courage, and practical tools, in addition to clear agreements between you and your partner.

Talk to your partner about your attractions and fantasies instead of acting them out… Learn to manage attractions before they happen. Sit down with your partner and discuss what happens if one of you has an attraction to someone else and cheats. What are the consequences? These consequences should be labeled and very clear, so if one of you is tempted to cheat, they know exactly what they are risking.

In my opinion, people in developed countries respect the law because of the negative reinforcements/consequences of breaking the law. For instance, if you violate a traffic law, you will face a negative consequence such as wasting money on tickets and attorneys, going to jail, or having your license removed; this keeps most people behaving desirably by complying with traffic laws.

Each relationship is unique, so you and your partner should determine what is best for your relationship and each of you. What does be in an open or a closed relationship mean to you? (Chapter 7). Remember, everything is fine if it is consensual. Explore each other's boundaries, renew them, and make sure you don't cross lines. Then, you can prevent "the ghost." Being faithful is a choice, a decision you make. Dr. Helen Fisher—mentioned in the Introduction and in Chapter 2—well known for her studies on romantic love and author of many great books including *Anatomy of Love* says, "fidelity is not natural." So, you must work on it.

As a couple, Pedro and I have done exactly this. We proposed a model, the *Infidelity-Fidelity Model* to better deal with infidelity based on negative and positive reinforcement/consequences, where desirable behavior (fidelity) is strengthened by stopping, removing, or avoiding a negative outcome (consequences of betrayal), and reinforcing it positively when achieved. The consequences must be clear, severe, realistic, and considerably risky, because opportunities to cheat are all over. Opportunities—chances to be involved in risky situations where you can cheat—must decrease and/or be avoided, especially when alcohol or drugs are involved.

I believe that when you are strongly connected—sexually and emotionally—have established agreements, know the consequences of breaking those agreements, and have consciously reduced opportunities where you feel vulnerable to cheat, you may prevent infidelity—but this doesn't mean it is guaranteed; just better chances of keeping ourselves out of the slippery slope!

Our *Infidelity-Fidelity Model* consists of four specific variables: Opportunities, Connection (sexual and emotional), Agreements, and Consequences. Remember that fidelity is not natural; it is a conscious decision that requires some mental effort. This model shows how the minimization or maximization of these four variables promotes either fidelity or infidelity. Low opportunities, high consequences, high connection, and clear agreements contribute to fidelity. The opposite is also true and contributes to infidelity. Don't get me wrong, opportunities are great to grow and have novel experiences to keep your love life "alive" —as long as you experience them TOGETHER, without cheating and lying.

Please see the *Infidelity-Fidelity Model*, which I present below:

Infidelity-Fidelity Model

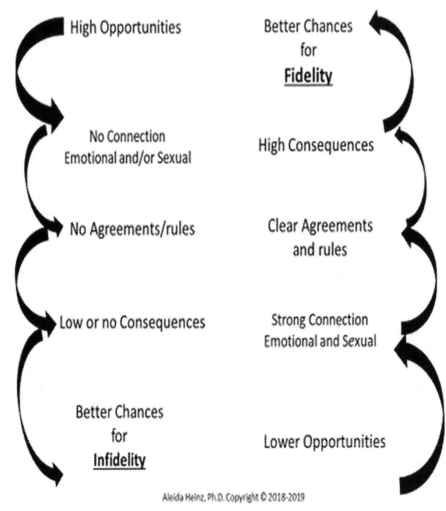

High Opportunities

Better Chances for **Fidelity**

No Connection Emotional and/or Sexual

High Consequences

No Agreements/rules

Clear Agreements and rules

Low or no Consequences

Strong Connection Emotional and Sexual

Better Chances for **Infidelity**

Lower Opportunities

Aleida Heinz, Ph.D. Copyright © 2018-2019

Infidelity-Fidelity Model

There is no way to guarantee your partner will not cheat. Nothing is guaranteed in life but death! So, don't be naïve about the possibility of infidelity. Do your best to prevent such a destructive behavior and the resentment that it brings.

Trusting Again

To be able to trust is wonderful! Trusting your partner is about the firm belief in the ability of your partner. It is about confidence, strength, certainty, and faith. If infidelity is an act of betrayal, the core of betrayal is that broken trust. Your trust in your partner has been broken, so to get it back, you must make it stronger than before…

I see trust as a space for uncertainty and ambiguity between partners where you choose to believe in the fulfillment of the agreements and promises you've made to one another. The hope you have in one another gives you comfort and safety. You cannot be 100% sure about your partner, and whether they will keep to your agreements, because you cannot be 100% sure about anything! You must have *faith* that your agreement will be honored. Create agreements to create trust.

If you think you are naïve, it is not because you trust too much. It's because you aren't communicating well. Naivety is being blind to uncertainties or concerns. Face issues, either from the past or those that could happen in the future. Don't wait for "the storm to destroy your home" —fix problems before they happen, as that is the only way you will be protected.

Building true intimacy and assertive communication (as discussed in the next chapter) are key and essential factors for repairing your love life. Keep in mind that the ultimate fidelity is to yourself. Be true to yourself, first and foremost, and then to your partner. Please get back to trust again and aim for the best possible feelings for your partner in order to make love again…and *make love 365 times a year!*

Part II: Another Inseparable Duo: Emotions & Feelings

So often in my practice, I hear the phrase: "I love my partner but…" What kind of love is that? When you say "but" it probably means that something is missing—your love is an incomplete type of love, so it is possible that you are only enjoying some aspects of love, not all. A deep exploration of your feelings is crucial to examine your emotional life in order to determine which feelings are positive and which are negative, why so, and when they started.

First, know that feelings and emotions are not the same. They are, however, highly connected, like hands and fingers, or brain and mind. One supports the other, influencing and determining what happens. Let's first differentiate feelings from emotions, then understand them and how they work.

Emotions and Feelings

Emotions are temporary reactions from an event that impacts our mood. They can be measured in physical ways—through brain scans or noticeable physical reactions, postures, or facial expressions. We smile when happy or cry when sad. You feel emotions in your body. This is just part of being human; emotions are universal. Even though emotions themselves are momentary, they can have a long-lasting effect, especially when they are repeated. This is doubly true if they are strong and powerful. On the other hand, feelings are more mental and stable. They are mental associations your brain makes from your emotional experiences. So, it works like this: you perceive and give meaning to your emotions, which become feelings.

First, you perceive the emotion you are experiencing through your senses, and then it travels to your brain. A mental association is created, so your feelings are based on the emotions you are experiencing and your interpretation of them. You're giving meaning to your emotions and creating new feelings or reinforcing existing ones.

Know that emotions are universal and can be measured, whereas feelings cannot adequately be measured and are not the same for everyone; they can be interpreted differently based on many factors. Different people can create different feelings from the same emotional event. Again, feelings, like the feeling of love, cannot be measured like emotions can. The feeling of love is an especially unique interpretation of emotion. What may be love for you is not necessarily love for me. This feeling is unique for everyone. Emotions are experienced in your body; feelings are stored and experienced in your mind. This is one of the main reasons I started with your mindset in Chapter 1, because in your mind you can store everything—and you need to be aware of that!

Your mindset helps you filter your emotions since the process is usually unconscious; you are not aware of these associations and feelings forming. For instance, if you have a weak, poor mindset about sex, then you don't have a conscious filter to get rid of any unpleasant, sex-related emotions. Without a strong mindset, you may create unconscious based on bad moments, which can skew your viewpoint.

Go ahead and work on your mindset if you haven't done so! Your strong mindset about love, sexuality, and your relationship must be set and ready as soon as possible for the future emotions in your life! Always remember that you cannot choose the emotions you will experience from future events, but you can choose how to perceive them in order to build positive feelings. And you perceive through your mindset!

Future emotions will be spontaneous and inevitable, and they will be associated, interpreted, and given meaning by your mindset to be stored as powerful feelings. So, your emotions unconsciously lead to feelings. These feelings then affect how you'll emotionally react to a situation. It's a cycle of emotions and feelings. If any issues are not treated, then this can turn into a vicious cycle.

It is all too easy for bitter emotions to lead to bitter feelings if filtered through a poor mindset. These bitter feelings will then cause poor actions that will lead to further bitter emotions and feelings, creating resentment. Being unaware of your resentment can lead you towards depression, anxiety, displeasure, and dissatisfaction in the bedroom. These can cause further harder feelings, which lead to—you guessed it—more negative emotions and feelings.

Remember, from Chapter 1, that, we often create our first mindset using other people's ideas, thoughts, beliefs, and experiences—our old paradigm. This creates a negative cycle that you must learn how to break. Why is this so important? If you are full of negative feelings toward your partner, it will be very difficult to connect. How can you *make love 365 times a year*? Sexual intimacy becomes almost impossible! Resentment and hard feelings bring difficulty and unhappiness, blocking your "route" to a fulfilling love life. Remember, your feelings toward your partner and your emotional connection are "the route" to lovemaking. Cleaning out your emotions is essential when looking to improve your sex life.

Dr. John Gottman, leading psychologist and founder of The Gottman Institute, states that "emotional disengagement is a dysfunctional pattern leading couples to divorce an average of 16.2 years after the wedding." In the Gottman Institute, couples learn to repair past hurts and increase closeness to deepen the emotional connection. This is what I do daily in my practice, helping couples reconnect emotionally and overcome past wounds, before assisting them to connect sexually. This is how I helped John and Alexa. I made them talk about the resentment they had. Alexa was finally able to express her emotional pain from the past—when she was pregnant—and was able to get rid of it. After that, they both were able to experience better feelings for each other.

Think of your first sexual emotion with your current partner. Go to the very beginning, when you were first forming feelings for your partner. More than likely, those first emotions were positive and led to good feelings. Now, think of the first negative emotion you've experienced with your partner, sexually or otherwise. If for any reason you experienced uncomfortable situations, producing negative emotions, you probably perceived them as hurtful—according to your mindset—and created unconscious negative feelings towards similar situations, or even toward your partner. These feelings will constantly create more negative emotions towards your partner or a situation, making you avoid them, which will lead to more negative feelings and reinforce the negativity.

What a terrible circuit!

Over time, all these negative feelings will worsen and get deeper; they don't disappear. On the contrary, more negative emotions will reinforce negative feelings, and it will become almost impossible to dissolve them in some cases. Instead, build and concentrate on the positive feelings you have for your partner and face resentment now! Today is the day, because if you don't face the trouble, then you will flee, avoiding the issue. As you avoid dealing with it, you and your partner will slowly settle but will be disconnected even more. This will only create more negative feelings such as fear, anger, sadness, and hatred.

A study done in 2013, published in the Journal of Marriage and Family Therapy, found that withdrawal behaviors—avoiding the issue—in a relationship predicted higher divorce rates and unhappiness. The same is true for couples engaging in demand/withdraw behaviors—one of them pressuring and receiving silence in return.

Daily life, in the form of work, children, housework, bills, and overall difficult situations, etc., if not handled well, can cause a lot of stress and negative feelings towards your partner. This will extend to your sex life and cause it to deteriorate before you know it. If you don't realize this, it could get worse and only cause resentment.

If you believe the myth that great sex is natural, then you won't put any work into sex. Great sex is not natural and negative feelings will keep you from initiating sex—or any physical contact with your partner. Don't be that naïve! Work must be put in for good sex to survive in any long-term relationship and working on your feelings is a big part of the work—an indispensable requirement—in order to *make love 365 times a year.*

Feelings and the Conditioned Negative Sexual Responses

Recall now from Chapter 2 the formation of conditioned negative sexual responses which contribute to sexual problems. As prominent psychologist Hans Eysenck says, "all neurosis is essentially conditioned emotional responses." After experiencing negative feelings, over and over, you will condition a natural response—a normal, positive, easy, spontaneous response—into a negative one.

For example, if the first time you ask about sex someone yells at you and tells you not to talk about it, that sex is dirty and bad, you may associate sex with yelling, dirtiness and shame. This will condition you to not talk about sex for fear of being yelled at. If someone mentions sex, you may immediately feel ashamed when talking about it, just like that first time. This is a conditioned negative response—Chapter 2. These conditioned negative emotions about sex can cause you to overreact in some situations with your partner, especially when sex is involved. Suddenly you have a certain view of yourself, based on these negative feelings: "I don't like sex." It's not that you don't like sex! It is that you don't like the unconscious emotions associated with sex: shame, guilt, anger, hatred, or/and disgust. And this is crucial.

Feel your feelings and confront them when you are with your partner, so you can know what your true feelings are. Without consciously acknowledging your feelings, you won't understand them. Maybe you have normalized negative feelings. Resentment doesn't come from thin air; it builds upon itself gradually. Only with a real, honest look at your feelings, by talking about them, and consciously describing them, will you be ready to let them go! That's what John and Alexa did.

If you are experiencing unpleasant sensations and emotions during sex, it may be due to conditioned negative responses that you are probably not aware of, blocking your path to sexual pleasure. All of this impacts your love life, which may become miserable. If your love life is a disaster, how will you have a good quality of life and *make love 365 times a year*? John and Alexa had an unpassionate love life because of their fears and resentment for each other.

Together they accumulated conditioned negative sexual emotions and feelings. This negativity is a passion killer! I see this case after case. Once a passionate relationship dies, it is hard to reignite it again—it's hard, but not impossible!

Restoring Positive Feelings

My three steps to creating better feelings are:

1. Awareness of feelings: Ask yourself questions related to your feelings for your partner, your relationship, and your love life. Face your negativity. Many people will indeed become workaholics, alcoholics, or childrenaholics—too centered around their children—to avoid conversations.
2. Understand where your feelings come from. Like we talked about before, go back to when you first met, and when you had your first negative reaction toward your partner. Women are more likely to be able to recall these events than men. But, together or separately, try to look back and see what happened.
3. Take action and improve your feelings! Now that you're aware of these feelings, learn to respond differently, especially in the bedroom. Cut the cycle by creating new, positive emotions together that will generate positive feelings toward each other. Create new positive responses.

These three steps sound simple, but they are very powerful. Using this skill, you can reset and begin fresh with new feelings. Think of it like this—if your vacuum breaks because the filter is full, you must empty it to make the vacuum work again. Your mind is the same way! There is limited space for all your feelings, so keep only the positive ones.

Remember how you started before, the excitement and thrill you got when you first began your sex life with your partner. Try to recreate these nice sensations again. To accomplish such a task, I will refer to the Italian term *Sprezzatura*, defined as the art of making something difficult seem easy and effortless, as if it were natural and simple—but it is not!

Sprezzatura means the accomplishing of difficult actions which require conscious effort in an "apparently" effortless way. So, embody it! Make the daily interactions between the two of you easy and effortless, at least by pretending in the beginning—sprezzatura—so that these interactions will eventually become truly easy and fun—because you have learned to enjoy them and have deconditioned yourself.

Little by little, your trust and desire for more will regrow. As you hold conversations with your partner, make sure to respond consciously rather than unconsciously, or automatically without thinking. So, THINK and FEEL. If you are inserting positive thoughts and feelings into your experience, then you can grow and re-learn.

Try to understand what your partner is looking for, and the best way to express your love. As Gary Chapman mentions in *The 5 Love Languages*, find your partner's favorite way to communicate loving feelings. What is your love language? Do you know your partner's love language? Love is a positive feeling that comes from emotions perceived as good and heartwarming. Make more feelings of love in your relationship every day to *make love 365 times a year.*

Dr. Albert Ellis, form Chapter 1, said that "people tend to function better when they are feeling better." If you consciously make yourself feel positive and calm, then you will be positive and calm in your love life. You have the power to control your feelings through your mind, by perceiving and interpreting your experiences and events in a suitable, favorable way.

Unpleasant emotions may happen in the future; you are still human. But if you understand how emotions work, and how they affect you and your partner, you will consciously manage them rather than just let them build up. Psychologist and sex therapist Dr. Jude Cotter, suggests that "a good sex life comes out of a good love relationship." Lovemaking requires good feelings. As Birch says, "sex, after all, is a physical expression of what's going on in a relationship."

Part III: Having Sex vs. Making Love

According to my findings, one of the key components for a successful sex life is to be able to distinguish between having sex and making love. But first, you should know that these are two different activities that are inspired by different chemical components in the brain and are performed for different reasons.

I have found that most people confuse the two concepts or are not clear about the terminology—sex versus lovemaking. Most people I interviewed believe that lovemaking is the romantic, passive, kind, soft, and even the "decent," "romantic," or "boring" version of sex—but this is incorrect. The big difference lies in the feelings of the participants and the purpose of these actions.

This chapter is mainly about lovemaking—the heart of this book—and the main idea is to explain the differences between sex and lovemaking. In this way, I can redefine concepts through facts and scientific evidence, show you the elements needed to sustain a passionate love life, and open the door to the realistic possibilities of *making love 365 times a year.*

Let's learn to make love as part of your healthy lifestyle! So, let me ask you the same two questions I asked many people in a survey. Think of—or better yet, write down—your immediate thoughts to these questions. So, grab a pen and paper, and feel free to write as much as you want.

Questions:

1. What do the words "sex," "having sex," or "fuck" mean to you? And, what are your first thoughts when you hear the following expressions?

   ▶ "I want you."
   ▶ "Let's do it now."
   ▶ "You arouse me."
   ▶ "You're so hot."
   ▶ "Let's have sex."
   ▶ "I want sex."
   ▶ "Want to eat you."
   ▶ "Want to have sex with you."
   ▶ "Want to fuck you."
   ▶ "Want to have sex."
   ▶ "Get down."

2. What do the words "love," "make love," or "lovemaking" mean to you? What are your first thoughts when you hear the following expressions?

   ▶ "I love you baby, let's make love."
   ▶ "Want to love your whole body."
   ▶ "Let's love each other."
   ▶ "Let me feel you."

Is there any difference in your thoughts, reaction, and answers to each of these questions? What do these statements, implicating sex and lovemaking, mean to you? What thoughts came to your mind? I want your own words and opinions on this. Once you've written down your answers, take a look. Did something change between "sex" and "making love?" What do your answers tell you?

I have asked these same questions to many men and women of different ages, cultures, race, and backgrounds, single or in a relationship. These are some of the answers I got for the first group of questions about sex:

- ▶ "Let's do it!"
- ▶ "Umm...sounds good to me."
- ▶ "It's all crazy and exciting."
- ▶ "Sex is adventurous, exciting, and fun to me."
- ▶ "Sex allows you to invent and make up, it's adventure."
- ▶ "Always something new to try."
- ▶ "Lust, lusty."
- ▶ "Orgasms! Cum, Coming."
- ▶ "Anywhere, anyplace! In the car, kitchen, out of the bedroom."
- ▶ "Take your clothes off."
- ▶ "Wanting to fuck, it makes me think of genitals."
- ▶ "Not if I'm tired."
- ▶ "I hate that expression; don't call it fucking."
- ▶ "I never say fuck when talking about sex."
- ▶ "That gives me anxiety; I don't like the word, don't know how to fuck."
- ▶ "The man becomes an octopus; he's touching me everywhere."
- ▶ "Doggy style."
- ▶ "Ass or anal play."
- ▶ "She's on top."
- ▶ "Having a quickie."
- ▶ "Whenever, whatever, anywhere, any place."
- ▶ "Get over."
- ▶ "Oral sex."
- ▶ "Wild, hot, pleasure, sweat, crazy, exciting."
- ▶ "For men and whores."
- ▶ "Individualistic."

I noticed that men seemed more excited by the idea of "sex" than women. Every woman I asked immediately got reserved, even if she later opened and said she enjoys sex.

Now, compare those answers to the ones I received when asked the second group of questions. These are some of the answers I got for the second group of questions about lovemaking:

Answers about lovemaking:

- ▶ "Missionary position, he on top."
- ▶ "Love and passion. Passionate."
- ▶ "Goofy."
- ▶ "Tender, nice and soft…romantic and passionate sex."
- ▶ That exists? The same thing as sex but more romantic."
- ▶ "Boring."
- ▶ "Repetitive, slow, not much fun."
- ▶ "Non-adventurous. Boring!"
- ▶ "For committed people. Means commitment."
- ▶ "Intimacy."
- ▶ "It is a different mind-set."
- ▶ "Involves feelings…it moves me."
- ▶ "We are in a bed…in the bedroom."
- ▶ "There's foreplay."
- ▶ "It's soft, sweet, and tender version of sex."
- ▶ "We share it together."
- ▶ "Lots of kisses…surrender."
- ▶ "I have multiple orgasms."
- ▶ "It's complicated…I like it, but it is difficult."
- ▶ "I don't know what that is."
- ▶ "Playing with genitals."
- ▶ "It's like more work."
- ▶ "It's more from the mind."
- ▶ "It inspires me. It is beautiful."
- ▶ "A team effort."
- ▶ "There's love, music. It's slow and passionate."
- ▶ "There's communication. No dirty words."

Can you see the different responses and expectations for sex and lovemaking? It may get very confusing for most people. Psychologist Dr. Elliot D. Cohen, President of the Institute for Critical Thinking, affirms that "having sex, even great sex, is not necessarily making love....unfortunately, this common use (or misuse) of the terms—having sex vs. making love—can mask the important distinction between these two activities."

Having sex and making love are not the same. Even if the perceptions are different, some people still use the term lovemaking to soften "having sex," as we may see in the above answers. Most people think that making love is a euphemism for sex or see it as a sophisticated word for sex. They believe that sex and making love are almost the same thing, with some variations. This can be especially true for those with a religious background, who may believe lovemaking is a nicer term for sex.

But, by confusing these two terms, you can ruin your sex life! Why?!

Because you might create false expectation; for instance, when believing that someone is going to make love to you, when in fact they only want to have sex. Disappointment and frustration from the experience can be emotionally painful, generating unpleasant feelings toward being sexual. Keeping these two concepts separate, will help you have more realistic expectations.

Furthermore, if you are in a long-term relationship and still believe that the two terms—having sex and making love—are the same, you will not make any effort to improve your sex life and learn to make love. That is, you will wait just to have sex without concentrating on the love you feel for your partner.

Having Sex

Healthy sex is a physical expression and manifestation of your desires. It's an activity, an action, something you do with your genitals. It is a genital activity! Genitals play a leading role when having sex; usually they are the focus of your attention, and the main element at play.

Sex can be performed in many ways, from manual play to intercourse. In manual play you use your hands, fingers, and genitals, in oral sex you use your mouth and genitals, in anal sex you involve the anus, and in, in intercourse, you penetrate, or are penetrated. So, sex is not intercourse; remember that sex is everything you do with your genitals—sexual acts—including penis-in-vagina intercourse. No more, no less. One of the greatest myths and misunderstanding about sex is that it is equivalent to intercourse.

Sexologist, founder of the Northwest Institute on Intimacy, and author of *Sex, God, & The Conservative Church: Erasing Shame from Sexual Intimacy*, Tina Schermer Sellers, PhD, talks about this misconception of sex. She says, "it seems in the straight world when the word 'sex' is used the assumption is that penis and vagina intercourse is the topic…intercourse is the assumed definition of sex, and if intercourse does not happen, every kind of intimate touch that has transpired between she and her partner are negated…sex is not meant to be a transaction, it is meant to be a playful, pleasurable, desired co-constructed exchange of intimate touch between people." Cohen describes the act of having sex as "a mechanical activity…rubbing, touching, caressing, kissing, sucking, biting, and, of course, intercourse, as fulfillments of a desire for physical contact, are all sexual activities in this sense."

Normally, the purpose of healthy sex is to fulfill sexual urges, desires, fantasies, to give and receive pleasure, and for procreation. It is always about needs and sexual pleasure, about "me and my needs." Usually the main goal of having sex is to orgasm—to come—to become sexually satisfied. Woody Allen said it best: "Sex alleviates tension."

Sadly, in many cases in various societies, sex has been misused and abused in different ways—provoking all kind of negative reactions and feelings. Sex as a duty, as an obligation, as a wifely task, to get attention, to be loved, to control, to punish or reward, or to manipulate people, are typical examples of the misuse and abuse of sex, and it is more common than you might think.

This misuse of sex has been one of the biggest mistakes of society, turning this healthy activity—sex—into something negative, unwanted, shameful, tedious, boring, and even sick. Furthermore, sex is often wrongly confused with love and expected to fulfill emotional emptiness, leading to even more emptiness, loneliness, and confusion. Like most things in life, unhealthy sex has a spectrum of possibilities, from being boring to violent or even criminal. Whether through the scope or the scale, these unhealthy sexual activities are detrimental to your well-being and to your sexual happiness.

We need to update the concept of marriage and relationships to understand that no one owns anyone! A wife is not her husband's property, and vice versa. Your partner doesn't belong to you, you both belong to a relationship. As I say to my couple clients, *my client is your relationship*—not one of you or the other. In this way, the solution to improve things should be based on what is good for "our" relationship, rather than what is good for "me."

Furthermore, being in a relationship doesn't give you the right to coerce your partner to have sex whenever you want. Sex is not, and never should be, one more "duty" to do. If sex is felt as an obligation or something you "supposed to do", it will only bring anxiety, fear, disgust, and even hatred. As Schermer suggests, "obliterating women's natural desire to be sexual."

Sex is a non-reciprocal activity, since commonly people are most focused on their own pleasure and needs. Even if your pleasure is to please, it's still about your need to please. On many occasions sex is not enjoyed reciprocally, it is not a mutual activity; that is, not all participants are having the same fun, and/or each one is lost in his own world of pleasure and fantasy. So, sex is mostly self-oriented; it is not about loving you, it is about wanting you…about "fucking you."

On top of that, sex doesn't need love to be great. Love isn't a requirement for sex, even amazing, mind-blowing sex! There is no single sexual activity that requires love. It does not mean that having sex is inferior than making love—it's just different. But, making love does require love!

Making Love

Lovemaking isn't just about having healthy and/or romantic sex; it is a lot more than that. Lovemaking is the ultimate expression of love and the ultimate way to deeply connect as a couple. As I said before, to have sex, even great sex, you don't need love, but to make love you do. Love is the fundamental ingredient of lovemaking. Without mutual love, you can have great sex, but can't make love. It seems obvious, but in my opinion, most people don't realize it.

Furthermore, Love & Connection is one of our fundamental human needs that must be fulfilled for our overall well-being. And, what a great way to fill that need: *making love 365 times a year*! In fact, when love enters into the sexual equation—participants start loving each other—sex then is transformed into lovemaking. Lovemaking isn't only about what you do sexually, but how you feel towards your partner. In other words, it is not only about what you do but how you feel from now on.

When you are making love, your attention is no longer mainly focused on the genitals, as in the case of having sex—it is on the whole person, inside and outside, including minds, hearts, and souls, along with the genitals. The activity isn't self-oriented anymore, but a mutual activity, because now it is about "us"—sharing the same love, desire, and with the same energy and intention.

Hence, lovemaking goes beyond sex and orgasm. It is the ultimate body-heart-mind-soul pleasure with the main purpose of connection. Orgasm is a great bonus which should occur as a result, not as a goal or requisite. Again, to stay deeply connected is your reason for *making love 365 times a year,* not to orgasm 365 times a year... If that happens, great! But if not, that's also great.

When making love, maybe you will experience orgasm, maybe only your partner, maybe both of you will or neither of you will, and that's still okay. Just enjoy the pleasure of feeling each other and the opportunity to be together as lovers...with no pressure or expectations. In that way, you will not have to be guided by your physiological needs—like most animals are—but by your decision, desire, and willingness to connect and remain connected to your partner through the pleasure of lovemaking... In other words, it should be the love for each other that motivates you to be sexually intimate and not your sexual needs...

Love is about trust, honesty, openness, independence, and surrendering to each other in healthy ways. So, what does *love* have to do with hormones, age, physical condition, work, Netflix, viruses, social distance, or being tired? These are reasons I hear all the time that prevent couples from intimate touching.

Be aware then that lovemaking is always healthy and pleasurable, as love should be. There isn't room for coercion, force, threat, intimation, lies, manipulation, or obligation—as in the case of unhealthy sex. In fact, "unhealthy lovemaking" does not exist. Sex is selfish. True lovemaking is always compassionate. Sex only requires at least one hot body. Lovemaking requires two people full of love for each other in a respectful way.

Loving partners create emotional and sexual intimacy (discussed in the next chapter), and the willingness to keep loving each other throughout time. Understand that lovemaking is in no way a duty, a job, or a way to "get through sex." It is something you will truly want to do *365 times a year.* So, never forget that the main purpose of making love is connection and pleasure. Sexual satisfaction is "almost" guaranteed only if both of you have only the expectation of enjoying each other's love. Orgasm, as I said before, is a nice outcome, but the real experience transcends sexual pleasure; it is a soul pleasure!

Paulo Coelho, outstanding writer and author of *Eleven Minutes,* wrote beautifully what it means to make love, as I quoted at the beginning of this book: "Anyone who is in love is making love the whole time, even when they're not. When two bodies meet, it is just the cup overflowing. They can stay together for hours, even days. They begin the dance one day and finish it the next, or—such is the pleasure they experience—they may never finish it."

Lovemaking isn't about one; it's about two people being one. As Cohen says, "in lovemaking, there is a mutual consciousness of unbounded unity without partition…back to one of my favorite quotes by Aristotle, love is composed of a single soul inhabiting two bodies. You follow and are followed by your partner. There is an authentic unity, an element of respect, and reciprocity. Foreplay builds until two separate beings become one."

What fabulous quotes about lovemaking! Don't you want to know more?

More About Lovemaking

Know that when you are making love, you are choosing to express your love. That's it! It's a conscious decision to be unified and connected to one another. It isn't about control but about surrender. It is the ability to lose yourself in the other, as your partner loses themselves in you. It is all about feeling each other, over and over… So, wake up your feelings of love to *make love 365 times a year.* Negativity won't let you surrender, connect, and freely enjoy your partner.

Unity, authenticity, mutual respect, appreciation for each other, no sacrifices, no denial of self, free will, no expectations, play, intimacy, solidarity, and a deep connection are what make two differentiated people become one united in pleasure and sensations to make love.

As I stated in the introduction, the idea of this book is to provide you with some reliable tools, which I have found necessary for a healthy sex life, so that you can *make love 365 times a year.* When I say, "to make love" or "lovemaking," it means having healthy sex with feelings of love for each other. It will never be the intention of this book to promote irresponsible, unhealthy, or risky sex, by any means. This is not a race to fuck a lot in a year, or to keep a number; it is about experiencing romantic love every day, a path to grow together, deeply connect, and have intense pleasure.

Having Sex or Making Love? How to Know?

Sex with intimacy, lust, desire, pleasure, and passion is *great sex.* Sex with intimacy, lust, desire, pleasure, passion, AND love is *lovemaking.* Now, can pure sex become lovemaking? Or, can lovemaking become just sex?

Absolutely! Yes, both cases are possible.

While having sex can become lovemaking over time, the opposite is also true. Many times, over the years, two people having great sex may fall in love, and sooner than later, they start loving each other, thus they start making love.

Remember, when love enters the equation, you are no longer just having sex, you are both making love. And I mean both—it takes two to tango!

On the other hand, lovemaking can turn into plain sex when, for example, negative emotions get in the middle. That is one of the reasons why communication is so important (discussed in the next chapter) because you don't want hard feelings and resentment to build up and destroy your love life. Then, you will no longer make love; you will occasionally have some sex, "if you are lucky..." but no lovemaking.

Healthy great sex is fantastic, but realistically, having great sex with high frequency is, for most couples, extremely difficult to sustain over the years, especially in ripe age in a long-term marriage. Many couples try to do this— trying to push themselves to have great sex to keep their sex life—but the frustration of not being able to sexually perform regularly discourages them to the point of avoiding sex—all or nothing. Consequently, anxieties and fears arise which will eventually disconnect you.

On the other hand, that is not the case for lovemaking. As I said, lovemaking is about love and connection rather than sexual performance. In this sense, you can sustain it over time, even in ripe age, with a high frequency, because you are not complying with the demands of great sex—which mostly depends on sexy context, sexual desire, arousal...

Always remember that you can have great, healthy and pleasurable sex without love, but you cannot make love without love...

Understanding Love to Make Love

There is plenty of scientific evidence to prove that love actually exists. Love is not an emotion; it is a deep, lasting feeling, as I explained in Part II. And, to make love, you need to understand the feeling of love.

According to Dr. Ellis, "love is created when you evaluate something (or someone) in a strong positive manner, that is, perceive it as being good, beneficial or pleasant... Love is an exceptionally good antidote for all kinds of fears; and to the extent that we have little love, we tend to have more fear, including sex fear." Therefore, love exists and is a powerful positive energy that overcomes any fear. Where there is love, there is not fear...

The Chemistry of Love

In the 80's, psychiatrist Michael Liebowitz proposed two phases in romantic love: Attraction and Attachment. In the 90's, anthropologist Dr. Fisher—mentioned before—proposed four phases and described the brain chemistry involved in each phase. The four phases are:

1. Attraction: The arousal phase—Pheromones
2. Infatuation: The in-love phase—Dopamine & Serotonin
3. Commitment: The love phase—Oxytocin & Vasopressin
4. Detachment: The "all is gone" phase—Cortisol (though we want to prevent this phase!)

Phase 1: Attraction: The desire and arousal phase. During this first phase of attraction, two people experience feelings of attraction and want to initiate something with the other person, maybe sex or a possible relationship. This phase is pure chemistry! The attraction is the phase of sexual gratification driven by testosterone, estrogen, and pheromones. Your brain will be releasing and producing these chemicals at a high rate. It is when you first want to be with "that" person, who you desire and are aroused by. The lust element comes into play as well as sex—lust and sex.

The brain is programmed for attraction, so around 50% of its focus (spontaneous focus, or attention) will be on exploring that "new" person that has attracted you, which does not mean being in love. Be aware that this process is spontaneous, easy, and natural. Once the new person becomes "not new" anymore, this process will no longer be spontaneous; you will need to put some effort into paying attention. Remember that!

Now, if you continue to be interested in that person; that is, you decide to voluntarily act on that attraction and have sex, you are going to intensify attention, so that attraction will become infatuation, which is an intense but short-lived passion and admiration for that person. Then, you may fall in love! That means that falling in love is really a decision made after acting on the initial attraction. So, if you decide not to "act on" that attraction, you probably will not fall in love.

Attraction, attention, and infatuation are crucial not only to fall in love, but to maintain the passion in any long-term relationship. As Fisher suggests, "don't copulate with people you don't want to fall in love with, because indeed you may do just that."

Phase 2: Infatuation: The in-love phase. It is the phase for intense, passionate love. The focus and the attention are all on one person (the key signal that you're in love with), so you become highly motivated. It is the motivational phase where you want to do everything possible to become better and pursue your dreams—if it is a healthy love. Then, you have fallen in love! You are now with a new person in a new relationship. You are now fully acting on these desires you felt in the attraction phase. The passion element comes into play—passion.

Your brain is filled with dopamine and serotonin, two of the most powerful and amazing neurochemicals. You are becoming fully aware and in love with this person. Your feelings are obsessive and intense; you are only feeling, with very little thinking. Dopamine is essential to feel love, for pleasure and *concentration*—focus. And that is exactly what you are doing in this phase: concentrating on that person and having pleasure! During this phase, you probably will experience great sex.

Now, if you stay in the relationship and continue to be interested in that person, thinking of a potential future with that person, your infatuation will become a commitment. You suddenly will be committed to that person, forming a stable relationship: the next phase!

Phase 3: Commitment: This is the certainty phase. It is where you find stability, continuity, and agreements. You are in a relationship! You can now relax. Normally, you experience a drop in dopamine and serotonin, but you will now release two more amazing neurochemicals: oxytocin and vasopressin—the attachment hormones. Recent studies have shown the correlation between levels of oxytocin and vasopressin and fidelity. Yes! We want that. Due to these wonderful hormones' production, your commitment may last without the "ghost of infidelity."

There are specific actions you can implement as daily love habits to release attachment chemicals, which are so important for keeping your connectivity. One of my favorites: "Pretzel Time," as I call it. Remember, it is a morning exercise for couples. As soon as you wake up, hug your partner as if you were a big pretzel. Stay there for at least 10 minutes as one delicious pretzel, very tight, naked, feeling and smelling each other! This is a simple but powerful way to release oxytocin and vasopressin to keep you connected through the day!

Oxytocin is the main connecting hormone that brings peace, calm, trust, fidelity, safety, and harmony in your relationship. You now have a sense of connectivity with your partner where you feel safe and attracted to this person. Only now is lovemaking possible. You start loving each other—love and intimacy.

This phase is wonderful. It is all you need to *make love 365 times a year*: attraction, desire (lust and sex) feeling in love (passion), connection, stability, safety, and commitment (love and intimacy). However, there is a risk during this phase that I want to warn you, and this is the familiarity that is generated from feeling too comfortable with each other. Be aware that your partner is still "your partner" rather than a good friend or a family member... That is why it is so important to know a bit about romantic love and to remember how things started: with lust, desire, and passion... If you stop *paying attention* to your partner and let the familiarity grow, your romantic love can be transformed into another type of love: a "friendship, roommate type of love."

Phase 4: Detachment: It is when you lose your love, your passion, and your relationship. Either through breakup or divorce. Cortisol is the chemistry in charge now—not good! The body may experience intense pain, there is no room for desire and pleasure anymore.

Why does detachment happen? According to my knowledge, it happens for one of these two reasons:

1. Poor mate selection. It was a wrong choice from the beginning: such a person—your partner or ex-partner—never was right for you in the first place, so it was an inevitable outcome. In this case, good for you! Most likely you fell in love with the wrong person, and in the third phase of commitment, where your eyes and your conscience opened, you realized you made a mistake! Probably your relationship will fail, and you will feel detached and disconnected. You then will enter in this last phase: detachment. As Fisher says, "who you choose matters."

2. Poor or no maintenance: You and your partner were not able to maintain the relationship in good shape, and instead neglected it. The positive behaviors that kept your relationship alive, and the reinforcements of your love life, are all gone. Familiarity, routine, domestic tasks, work,

duties, and stress prevent couples from enjoying romance, passion, and intimacy leading to disconnection and emotional/sexual ruin. The question is now how to maintain the fire, the lust, the desire, the trust, and all the right chemicals in your love life.

Now you can see that each phase has different neurological chemistry, so you feel differently, do different things, and act in different ways, according to your phase. Attraction leads to sex, which leads to attention. Attention leads to infatuation, leading to falling in love. Infatuation and falling in love lead to commitment and love.

There is more to learn about love, such as the types of love, and why you feel the way you feel about your partner. Why, in some cases, you are unable to make love to your partner, and why you can love two or more people at the same time.

Types of Love

Seven types of love have been identified by renowned psychologist, member of the Psychology Department at Yale University, and author of *The Triangle of Love: Intimacy, Passion, Commitment*, Dr. Robert Sternberg. Within these types of love lies an entire landscape of unique feelings which can help you differentiate the way you love.

According to Sternberg's triangular theory of love, these types of love are crafted out of three different components: intimacy, passion, and commitment. All THREE of these components are needed for a complete, mature, and healthy love. That is, intimacy, passion, and commitment are all essential to create a fulfilling relationship. But this is not always the case.

Sternberg clarified that "the amount of love one experiences depends on the absolute strength of these three components, and the type of love one experiences depends on their strengths relative to each other." These seven types of love are combinations of one or two of these three elements: passion, intimacy, and commitment.

You may be enjoying just two, or only one of these elements, but that means your love is incomplete—for instance, just passion (lust) is simply Infatuation. Just intimacy and commitment (feelings of love) are a Companionate love type—the common "roommate style." Just commitment is the Empty love type. And just intimacy and passion, without commitment, are the well-known Romantic love type.

It is important to be aware of the distinct types of love in order to know your love type. Without all three of these components—intimacy, passion, and commitment—there is no love at all, so it could be impossible to truly make love.

Let's look at the seven types of love according to these combinations—and sex.

1. Friendship love: There is only intimacy between you (there may be sporadic sex).
2. Infatuated love: There is only passion (there may be frequent great sex).
3. Empty love: There is only commitment— "the roommates" — (there may be little or no sex).
4. Romantic love: There is only intimacy and passion— "the 'lovers" — (there may be great sex or some lovemaking).
5. Companionate love: There is only intimacy and commitment— "the passionless friends" — (there may be some lovemaking with no passion).
6. Fatuous love: Passion and commitment only (predominantly great sex).
7. Consummate or Complete love: There is passion, intimacy, and commitment— "the fulfill couple" —it possesses all the ingredients (there may be *lovemaking 365 times a year...*).

There is nothing more wonderful than complete love in a long-term relationship. But, when someone only enjoys one or two elements in a relationship, then something is missing (which may make them go looking for it). We all need these three elements to feel fulfilled. This explains why it is possible to love more than one person at a time—but in different ways. The ideal is to have all the elements in one relationship.

In a Complete type of love, you can fulfill all your human needs. You can be yourself and trust each other (intimacy and connection), desire each other all the time (passion and uncertainty) and be trustful and stable (commitment and certainty). As Fisher said, "love is the most powerful sensation on earth."

If you love someone, then there is respect and admiration for each other; you both feel safe and secure, and can explore, play, and experience pleasure. Deep attraction and intense feelings over time occur when all these elements meet in one place—your relationship!

Do you understand a little bit more about love?

Sustaining Passion

Is it possible to sustain passion, lust, and desire over time? Yes! It is possible but with effort! You can learn to believe it is all new and unique in your relationship, so your brain will believe it too!

For decades, it has been thought that all committed couples, after a certain time of living together, inevitably cease to be in love, losing passion and lust—or replacing passion with a calm and relaxed love. Nowadays, new studies support the fact that long-term couples can remain in love over time, maintaining passion and lust for each other, and at the same time remain stable and committed.

One of these studies was done by Bianca Acevedo, PhD, and Arthur Aron, PhD, of the Department of Psychology at Stony Brook University. They used functional Magnetic Resonance Imaging (fMRI) to scan the brain of long-term happily married individuals (phase 3) and individuals who have recently fallen in love (phase 2). The results show that both groups have similar activity in a specific part of the brain.

That means, both groups—the ones in long-term happy relationships, and those recently in love—show similar neural activity in the ventral tegmental area (VTA) of the brain, as well as the substantia nigra. The study suggests that, "these brain regions are the clue to why some couples remain in love for years, even decades as if they were newly coupled."

Drs. Acevedo and Aron say, "there might be specific brain mechanisms by which romantic love is sustained in some long-term relationships." Furthermore, Acevedo and Aron suggested that "early-stage love can last through long-term relationships by engaging the rewards and motivation systems of the brain." The results revealed many other fascinating findings, uncovering some keys to maintaining lasting passionate love. One of them is focused attention! Remember, something you do spontaneously when you meet someone "new."

So focused attention is one of the main characteristics, found in both groups—newly in love and in love long-term—to preserve passion. Other studies done in the 2000's have also suggested that focused attention is key to maintaining passion in long-term relationships.

I know this is true! I am experiencing it in my own love life. We pay attention to each other every day, not in a spontaneous way as we did at the beginning of our relationship, but in a conscious way now—because we are no longer "new." So, you too can choose to pay attention to your partner and keep the passion in your relationship.

Isn't that amazing?!

Neuroscientist, psychiatrist, brain-imaging expert, and author of *Change your Brain Change your Life*, Dr. Daniel Amen found that "the brain is constantly seeking to keep itself balanced through increasing and decreasing the amount of these substances"—the neurochemicals in the brain. So, your brain needs to be balanced and keep a certain amount of all these substances—such as dopamine, testosterone, serotonin, oxytocin, vasopressin, among others—to properly work for you.

It is a constant balancing of dopamine (lust) and oxytocin, Vasopressin (love and intimacy). An amazing cocktail of dopamine, pheromones, oxytocin, and vasopressin to maintain your love life in good shape for many years! I want to get drunk with this super cocktail!

In my opinion, staying permanently fixed in one phase—usually phase 3, commitment (as you are meant to)—but experiencing only affection and caring, is not enough to keep your sex life in good shape—you need passion— because your brain will look for other elements for balance— for example, dopamine, which is easily obtained through infatuation. If you don't find this in your relationship, you'll find it somewhere else...

Again, it is about the constant balancing of lust, intimacy, and love to sustain passion. This information is fantastic to me, since unhappy couples can overcome the darkness of loneliness and the sadness of sexual disconnection due to their passionless relationships.

What else can you do?

Dr. Schwartz—form Chapter 2—conducted a study on extremely happy couples. Her study revealed five affective and effective behaviors that extremely happy couples around the world do as part of their routine. These habits, according to the study, kept these happy couples "passionately attached." These five common affective behaviors are:

1. Holding hands
2. Spontaneous kissing
3. Cuddling
4. Public displays of affection
5. Pet names

Easy and simple things to do, just like the Pretzel Time, to keep your passion and stay connected. So, please add these five behaviors plus Pretzel Time to your love equation! With all this valuable and updated information, I have made my own "love cocktail" to *make love 365 times a year.* The ingredients of my "love cocktail" are sex, love, lust, intimacy, and passion. I have called this love cocktail: LOVEX, which I will discuss and share with you next.

Part IV: The LOVEX Model

LOVEX is a concept that I have crafted and created to understand what is needed to make love. LOVEX is based on three recognized models of romantic love: Dr. Fisher's Theory of the Neurochemistry of Love, Dr. Robert Sternberg's Triangular Theory of Love, and Dr. Jack Morin's Love-Lust Model. Morin was a nationally known psychotherapist, sex therapist, author of *The Erotic Mind*, and a great professor of Human Sexuality—mentioned in Chapter 1.

The concept of LOVEX combines these three models, giving life to a more complete and more profound way of making love. It is about a new model that combines five elements—sex, love, lust, intimacy, and passion—to form a unity called LOVEX. So, when these five elements are harmoniously integrated and combined, LOVEX emerges, which will allow you to *make love 365 times a year.*

These five elements can and should work together in an entwined manner, with different intensities, shapes, and variations, to bring you a new and refreshing way to experience lovemaking. Lovemaking, then, can never be the same; the form and the intensity of these elements vary every day! Therefore, where there is LOVEX, there is no boredom, no obligation, performance, no emptiness. LOVEX is always pure, enjoyable, fun, pleasurable, emotional, hot, fulfilling, passionate, calm, and, above all, healthy.

Let's see why LOVEX is so amazing for your love life, according to these three outstanding models:

1. Dr. Fisher's Model: Refers to the chemistry of love, giving importance to love, lust, sex, intimacy, and passion—the components of LOVEX:

   Attraction: The arousal phase—pheromones (sex, lust)
   Infatuation: The In-love phase—dopamine and serotonin (passion)
   Commitment: The love phase—oxytocin and vasopressin (love, intimacy)

2. Dr. Sternberg's Model: Refers to the fundamental elements for a complete type of love, giving importance to intimacy, passion, and commitment—some of the components of LOVEX:

   Intimacy (intimacy, love)
   Passion (passion, lust, sex)

3. Dr. Morin's Model: Refers to the need for a balanced combination of love and lust for a healthy erotic sex life, giving importance to love and lust—the components of LOVEX:

   Love (love, intimacy)
   Lust (lust, sex, passion)

Now, let's see these five fundamental elements interacting as LOVEX to *make love 365 times a year:*

Love: encompasses attachment, care, attention, and positive feelings, so that you want to be as close as possible to your beloved. It is about "you," about your partner…the "I love you." About you caring for your partner's pleasure.

Lust: encompasses desire, fire, hotness, sexual sensations, attraction, wanting. The "I want you…" dirty games, fantasies, a vivid imagination, curiosity, seduction and eroticism.

Intimacy: encompasses honesty, openness, communication, conversations, closeness, vulnerability, and mutual understanding.

Sex: encompasses action! It is about "me," about my pleasure, the body, ecstasy…

Passion: encompasses intensity, energy, strong feelings of excitement and desire for each other. All the feelings and emotions together on a high level, strong, controllable, and very intense, driving you towards your partner. It is enthusiasm for your beloved, a fearless giving! Passion implies wild feelings and sharing an eager interest and curiosity.

Recent studies suggest that both passion and love encourage relationships well-being. As Oprah Winfrey once said, "passion is energy!" Sex without passion won't last; it may get very boring. Sex, love, lust, and intimacy with passion are endless, you'll share a synergetic pursuit to make love—love is also involved, it's not just great sex. It is about "us"—you and your partner *making love 365 times a year.* It is about "our" pleasure! I believe long-term couples need the combination of these five elements for great lovemaking.

A perfect dose of love and intimacy will bring you: care, security, stability, trust, certainty, pleasure and satisfaction. A perfect dose of lust, passion and genital interaction—sex —will bring you: desire, uncertainty, variety, curiosity, pleasure, and sexual satisfaction. Be aware that these doses vary according to your moods and contexts, but if all of them are present, *especially love,* you will be making love over and over in different and pleasurable ways—like the way you eat, from a little sandwich to a 5-star restaurant dinner—always something different, but you always eat! To experience lovemaking pleasantly, focus on the *love* that you feel for each other; the other elements will follow in different degrees, in each experience—in each "meal."

Morin says that "one of the key challenges of erotic life is to develop a comfortable interaction between our lusty urges and our desire for an affectionate bond with a lover, a bond that combines tenderness and caring with passion. Erotic health is possible as long as some degree of love-lust interaction exists at least some of the time." I have concluded that with good feelings and intentions in your hearts (love) that allow you to trust and open yourselves (intimacy) to your sexual desires (lust) to freely navigate each other's bodies (sex) to intensely experiencing (passion) the ultimate pleasure of a deep connection lovemaking. LOVEX to *make love 365 Times a year*! It can really heal and transcend you…

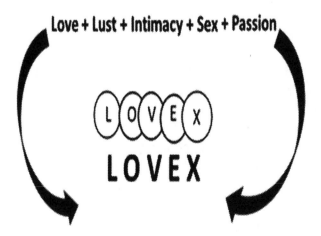

Love + Lust + Intimacy + Sex + Passion

LOVEX

Aleida Heinz, Ph.D. Copyright © 2019

The LOVEX Model

Now, how are you going to make this happen in a society that perceives lust, sex, and passion in a judgmental way? How are you going to integrate LOVEX in your love life? Let's examine that.

Creating LOVEX

Communication is key to creating LOVEX in your love life. Start by initiating conversations with your partner regarding each of these five elements—sex, love, lust, intimacy and passion—and what each one means to both of you.

Both of you need to know what is expected and what is possible. Men are usually good at describing sex but have more trouble with the idea of expressing love. Women usually struggle with articulating exactly what they want out of sex but are commonly pretty good about expressing feelings. And if your partner refuses to either talk about sex or feelings of love, then you need to know why. Learn to listen and express yourself. I will talk about expression and communication in the following chapter, because it is an important prerequisite to creating LOVEX in your life, in order to *make love 365 times a year.*

Likewise, if your partner is unable to speak, making love, or is not emotionally available, you should know that and take action now. If one partner can't make love due to emotional blockages or unavailability, there will be a conflict between you, ruining your sexual happiness. Seek professional help. Being willing and available is crucial for lovemaking.

It could be that a person—for instance, your partner—is unable of lovemaking because he or she has had traumatic experiences or unpleasant encounters in the past, or has used sex only to get attention, either to fulfill a false stereotypical ideal or to feel confident. Those who have been victims of sexual abuse usually express that, for them, sex has been detached from love and romance. So, it is essential to address this issue if any of these are the case. Don't just ignore or deny the pain that sex is causing you or your partner—seek professional help as soon as possible because you deserve to make love.

The 2017 documentary Liberated: *The New Sexual Revolution,* shows the attitude single young adults often have regarding sex and love, an extreme acting out of sexual desires to the point of sexual abuse and crime—unhealthy sex. This new "hookup culture of casual sex," has taken sex for granted, or as a game, sometimes with no respect for others. A culture that has taken love out of sex! Taking love out of the sexual equation is fine—there is nothing wrong with that—if you just want to enjoy having sex. However, to make love, you need to integrate love into the sexual equation. So, first, be clear about what you want and what your partner wants.

Overcoming Sexual Trauma

If you are in a long-term relationship and want to make love more frequently, you must overcome traumatic sexual experiences. In fact, it is also true that lovemaking could heal sexual trauma. And, overcoming those traumatic experiences is essential to create LOVEX.

According to The White House Council on Women and Girls, "one in five women is sexually assaulted while in college," most likely, creating sexual trauma. I see in my practice the dire consequences of trauma and sexual abuse and how this negatively impacts sexual pleasure. Have you ever thought about what will happen to those young girls who were victims of sexual abuse? How will their sex lives be as grown adults? Usually miserable, if they left the trauma unsolved, according to my professional experience.

Committed couples in long-term marriages are suffering today from "sexless relationships" in which they have sex ten times per year or less, according to recent researches. In my practice, I observe that lovemaking is not the norm for most married couples in the U.S. Some don't even know what lovemaking truly is; most long-term couples don't think about it. What is going on in this great country—and around the world? Dr. Ellis, mentioned in Chapter 1, wrote in *Sex without Guilt In the 21st Century* that "the vast majority of Americans experience a love life that is remarkable for its mediocrity." Why is that?

From my point of view, individuals go from "overly-sexed" when single, to "sexless" when married, and this shift is not healthy. A lot of sex with the wrong people and at inappropriate times, and years later, quite the opposite—very little sex with the right person, to whom you have chosen to spend your life, and in the appropriate time. Our societies are missing the beauty of sharing sexuality in all its aspects, including lovemaking. Sex has been reduced to a mere "simplistic genital act" with no essence. For victims of traumatic sexual experiences, a healthy sex life can be a hell of a lot of work. This is when lovemaking, not just sex, may become a healing power, to shift sex back to love and romance to trust again.

Well-known sex therapist and author of *Sexual Healing*, Barbara Keesling, PhD, tells us that "an intimate sexual relationship offers an excellent context in which we can experience the healing powers of touch. It appears that being touched in intimate areas taps into intimate thoughts and feelings; done from the heart, with honest openness, and without manipulative intent. An emotional bond cannot be forced, but it can be given the opportunity to grow."

What a powerful and wonderful message for all those who suffer and want to overcome the pain of bad experiences of the past... Now, the next step is to build LOVEX through communication and meaningful conversations with your loved one.

> "Start trusting and stop overthinking. Stay loyal to your dreams and have faith in the process. It's going to be worth it. One day you're going to be glad you never gave up despite facing challenges, setbacks, and heartache."
>
> —Vex King

Part V: 7 Suggestions & Recommended Sources

7 Simple Suggestions for Keeping Loving Feelings

1. Stay close to your partner, in the bedroom and out of the bedroom. Don't take your partner for granted. Go to bed together, at least most nights. Enjoy long, slow, non-orgasm-oriented lovemaking, without expectation, as much as you can. Make lovemaking a love habit, so, you can make love every day. Remember, you can make love the way you eat (from a simple sandwich to a fine dinner, you always eat!) Don't wait for your "libido," your libido—and desire—will follow you!

2. The challenge for every married couple is to stay CONNECTED. So, it is important to make a DAILY effort to do things together with affection, attention, awareness, and presence, so the feelings for each other can remain positive. Ask yourself the following questions:

   ▶ How do I feel when my partner touches me?
   ▶ How do I feel when I touch my partner? Do we touch each other?
   ▶ How do I feel when my partner speaks to me?
   ▶ How do I feel around my partner? Am I happier by myself?

> ▶ Do I want to spend time with my partner one-on-one?
> ▶ Am I using activities (work, kids, alcohol, phone, the Internet, etc.) to avoid talking with my partner?

3. Strengthen the emotional bond with your partner by creating a comfortable environment for deep communication, something important that most couples tend to neglect due to being "too busy." Good communication is essential to build trust, and trust is essential to make love. Avoid avoiding silence when things are not going well. Do not allow negative feelings build up to the point of "rotten fish." Don't build resentment!

4. As in our earliest childhood, we still need comfort when we feel hurt. Be that person for your partner; comfort him/her emotionally. We all have "bad" days, so be there for your partner without complain. Learn how to comfort and soothe each other and relieve any pain—physical or emotional—through your loving feelings to be able to make love.

5. Consciously pay attention to your beloved to avoid problems in your relationship. Remember that paying attention is easy at the beginning of a relationship when getting to know each other. As time passes, couples stop paying attention to each other. Staying fixed in the commitment phase—fulfilling your duties in the relationship/marriage—without romance, passion, and attention, means you aren't producing much dopamine.

6. You need to spice your relationship up through lust, romance, and focused attention. Seek out dirty, selfish, pleasurable, interesting, and novel experiences from time to time. Go LOVEX and be aware and keep working. Affectionate touch, tender love, and lusty feelings can always do magic in your love life; remain in love and in lust…

7. LOVE IS IMPORTANT—and LOVEX TOO! A recent study showed that small and deep parts of the brain such as the cingulate are activated in response to the sight—the face—of a romantic partner. So, activate such important areas in your brain by having pictures and photos of you and your partner in happy moments. Place an album in a place where you will frequently see it, like the kitchen or your bedroom. At least one

album with happy moments as a couple, only the two of you. It is not about a family album, but a romantic, sexy album.

8. Finally, if you don't have a partner, choose your next one well! Before forming a relationship, it is essential to make a good partner's SELECTION; that is, going through a process of selecting your mate and making sure you choose right and smart. As yourself these questions:

▶ What do I want?
▶ What kind of relationship do I want?
▶ Am I ready to give, receive, and share?
▶ How does my "ideal" partner look? What are they like?

Remember the first phase of Attraction. The attraction is pure chemistry; you don't choose to be attracted; you just are attracted to his/her pheromones. After that, THINK! The attraction is essential, but not enough on its own to form a healthy relationship. Before falling in love, think well and evaluate if that person is COMPATIBLE with you. That means their likes and dislikes, views of life, religion, spirituality, opinions on politics, sex, money, family, and so on.

I recommend you complete "my ideal partner check list" with your negotiable and non-negotiable areas. Also, your expectations in different areas such as physical, emotional, intellectual, sexual, social, political, and spiritual. Be as precise as possible, making a mental picture of the kind of person you want to live with.

This is the most important step, because the functionality of your relationship will depend on it. It is about THINKING before getting involved only by attraction. The greater the equality and knowledge about each other, the greater the success in the following phases. Studies indicate that compatibility, not compensation (opposites), best guarantees the most satisfactory and successful relationships. Mate selection is one of the most crucial and important decisions of your life. As Perel says, "the quality of our relationships determines the quality of our lives." So, think well before you fall in love with the wrong person.

Recommended Sources for Sex Secret #3

Sex without Guilt In the 21st Century by Dr. Albert Ellis

Change your Brain Change your Life by Dr. Daniel Amen

Emotional Intelligence by Daniel Goleman

The Erotic Mind: Unlocking the Inner Sources of Passion and Fulfillment by Jack Morin, Ph.D.

The Normal Bar: The Surprising Secrets of Happy Couples and What They Revel About Creating a New Normal in Your Relationship by Pepper Schwartz, Ph.D., et all

The Triangular Theory of Love by Robert Sternberg

Sexual Healing by Barbara Keesling, Ph.D.

The In-Factor Model: How the Internet Can Lead to Infidelity by Pedro Briceno, Ph.D., and Aleida Heinz, Ph.D.

The 5 Love Languages: The Secret to Love that Lasts by Gary Chapman

Are You Making Love or Just Having Sex? by Elliot D. Cohen

Anatomy of Love: A Natural History of Mating, Marriage, and Why We Stray by Helen Fisher, Ph.D.

Why We Love: The Nature and Chemistry of Romantic Love by Helen Fisher, Ph.D.

Liberated: The New Sexual Revolution documentary film by Dir. and Writ. Benjamin Nolot

The State of Affairs: Rethinking Infidelity by Esther Perel

Sex, God, & The Conservative Church: Erasing Shame from Sexual Intimacy by Tina Schermer Sellers, Ph.D.

Extraordinary Sex Now: A Couple's Guide to Intimacy by Sandra R. Scantling, Ph.D.

Me Aburrí del Sexo: Y Algunas Propuestas Tentativas para Salir del Aburrimiento by Rodrigo Jarpa Schacker (Spanish)

SEX SECRET 4

CHAPTER 4

Expressions

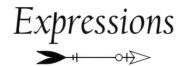

Life isn't only about survival; it's about living,
and so is making love.

—Mehek Bassi

Part I: Expressing Yourself

In my opinion, lovemaking is the most powerful *expression* of romantic love. On many occasions, sexual inactivity does not necessarily come from negative feelings, an unhealthy lifestyle, or a poor mindset about sex—it can be from not *expressing* your thoughts and feelings, from *repressing* them, or from *the way* you say things. Commonly, it is not what you say, but *how* you say it that might cause problems.

Little expression, poor communication skills, and lack of intimacy greatly affect couples, leading to disconnection, sexual apathy, and scarce lovemaking. You may love your partner and have nothing but positive feelings for them. But if you aren't communicating, there is still a problem—you aren't expressing your feelings at all. I know actions are important and show more than words, but expressions reinforce your actions, and may help you elaborate your feelings and thoughts and lead to closeness, especially for females—we are usually more auditory than males; usually we love to hear words of love and even that may arouse us.

Remember our analogy of the vehicle and route to explain what a fulfilling love life is. The GPS is our mind, the vehicle itself is our body, and the route is our feelings. Now, the next three chapters—Expression, Pleasure, and Eroticism—are about "the way" in which you want to travel. You can now ask yourself: how do I want to travel? Like it's a "race," or like a "pleasant journey?"

Before you choose, you need to pay attention to your environment, your context, your culture, and the culture you are in. These set your original paradigms and affect your actions. Your culture can determine what you'll do and the way you'll do it.

Let's take a look at new real cases—not just one, but three! Stephen and Valerie, Pasha and Kristen, and Richard and Jessica, three couples who, due to their poor way of communicating and expressing feelings, were almost led to sexual bankruptcy! Only the Lovemaking Wheels of the first couple will be shown (Case #4.1).

Case #4: Stephen & Valerie, Pasha & Kristen, and Richard & Jessica

Because this lack of intimacy is so common, this chapter has three real case examples. Lack of communication and intimacy is the number one problem I encounter in my practice. It does not allow a true connection, and if you are not connected, you can't *make love 365 times a year.* More than anything else, it is a couple's inability, or unwillingness, to communicate that leads to a "sexless" or non-sexual relationship. Let's review our cases:

Case #4.1: Stephen and Valerie: Stephen is 47, Valerie is 46, and they have been married for 14 years and have no children, which was a choice they made much earlier. They refer to one another as their "life-time partner." When they came to see me, they had been having very little sex for the past three years and were too fearful of discussing anything with each other, because they were worried about hurting each another's feelings.

As we were talking about feelings, I was able to observe their gestures and facial expressions of uncertainty, anxiety, and frustration. Through their expressions, I was able to understand how disconnected they were.

Case #4.2: Pasha and Kristen. This case is strikingly similar. Pasha is a 63-year-old male, and Kristen is a 58-years-old female. They have one child, age 20, and they also use the phrase, "life-time partner" when describing each other. When both couples approached me, they said the same thing when they sat down.

"We don't talk. We have NO communication."

Stephen claimed it was Valerie who wouldn't talk. "She's only black and white; the only communication I get is 'yes' or 'no.' She isn't talking! I need more information to be able to talk to her. She shuts down a lot. We don't talk, just watch TV, drink wine, and go out with friends."

Kristen had the same complaint of Pasha. "When we talk, the little we do say, I do not get anything from. He always been reserved, but now it is worse. I feel like I am just performing when we are in the bedroom. I do not understand him or what he wants anymore."

She looked shocked as she says the phrases I hear over and over. Her expression said it all.

"I don't know how we got to this point. We need to change."

Couples visit me because they realize they need to change their lives to enjoy a better sex life, and I'm sure that's also why you are reading this book. You realize something is wrong but have no idea what to do to fix it! But by recognizing there is a problem, you are taking the first step to fixing your love life. So many couples just accept that this is the way their lives must be. Stephen certainly felt that way, continuing to talk about what he didn't like about their current life.

"We are strangers!" he said. "We're together, but we don't talk. I feel like strangers living in the same house. We both have high libidos, but because we don't talk, we are no longer affectionate. We only have fun when others are around."

Kristen expressed a similar idea and said she couldn't figure out the problem. "I know he's not cheating," she said of Pasha. "But I don't know what he's thinking."

As always, I conducted individual interviews with each partner. I learned that in both of these couples, there was no cheating; they were just distracted and stuck. I saw they all loved their partner; there was no resentment, no fighting, no cheating, no hurt feelings. They were all physically active and had a good sexual mindset.

Stephen and Valerie just didn't know how to make love anymore. They were not expressing themselves, and when they did, they misinterpreted their desires. Kristen and Pasha were still far too interested in their son, who was living at home. They would only talk about the family business and their son's problems. They stopped talking about THEM: their feelings, their desires, the dreams they shared. They might have a great mindset about sex, but they had poor communication skills! While there was still love in the relationship, they didn't show it: no words, no affection, no touching. They no longer understood each other, causing disconnection and sexual inactivity.

Valerie didn't want to talk about sex, even about wanting it. "I don't know if he feels rejected and I don't want to know."

Kristen said something similar, but with her own problems. "I don't want to say what I want."

Pasha agreed. "I want to try and explore everything regarding sex. I have an open mind about everything. But I don't know how to talk to her."

"I don't know how to express anything," Kristen continued. "I feel disconnected because we don't talk, and we're not affectionate anymore."

Both couples knew they needed to communicate better, but they just didn't know how! Some couples have too many 'conversations': lots of fighting and, heated debates, or they won't leave each other alone. This kind of talking is also common, but these two couples are just the opposite. Now let's look at Valerie and Stephen's Lovemaking Wheels. Please, notice how low the expression element is for both:

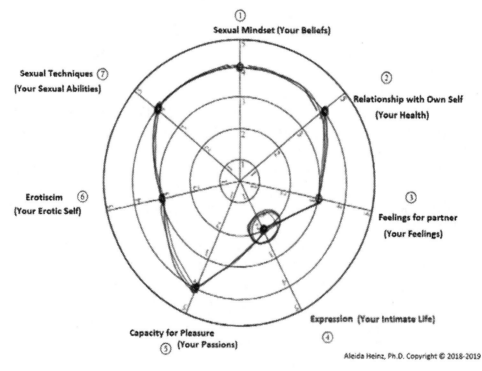

Valerie's Lovemaking Wheel. Wheel #7

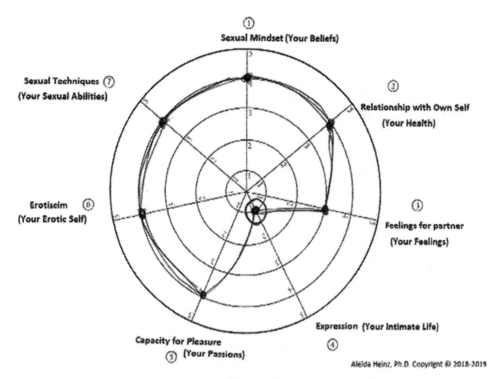

① Sexual Mindset (Your Beliefs)

⑦ Sexual Techniques (Your Sexual Abilities)

② Relationship with Own Self (Your Health)

⑥ Erotiscim (Your Erotic Self)

③ Feelings for partner (Your Feelings)

Expression (Your Intimate Life)

⑤ Capacity for Pleasure (Your Passions)

④

Aleida Heinz, Ph.D. Copyright © 2018-2019

Stephen's Lovemaking Wheel. Wheel #8

The third example I'd like to share with you is a bit unusual. It was about a man, Richard, that came to see me by himself in total pain. I felt as if his partner was there.

Case #4.3: Richard and Jessica. Richard was 42 and had been married to his wife Jessica, who was 37, for eight years. They didn't have any kids, and since Richard came to see me by himself, I never met Jessica.

"A lot is happening right now," he began. "I want to get divorced. I just don't know how to tell her."

"Why do you want to get divorced?" I asked. Most couples came to me because they wanted to avoid this!

"We have been together for fifteen years, and in the same situation that whole time. We're just contemplating the relationship, but we are afraid to talk."

"To talk about what?" I asked.

"To talk about how we don't talk!" he replied.

I asked Richard to tell me as much about his relationship as possible. Since

I never met Jessica, I never got her side of the story, but I tried to remain as neutral as possible while Richard talked.

"I'm tired of never talking," he explained. "We've never been passionate. We've been loyal, kind, and sweet. We're best friends. But we've never had a discussion! We don't communicate about our needs or desires. We just have sex sometimes. I enjoy sex with her, and I love her, but it's just sex. We've never talked about our dreams or our desires. No intimacy between us. We've never talked about anything painful. I can't feel satisfied with sex because we never talk about it after. She has an orgasm, I cum, and we go to sleep. That's it."

"I want to divorce her because I feel dead inside," he continued.

What did he want me to help him do? I wondered.

"My goal is to have our first real life conversation," he admitted.

He was nervous because even though he was very highly educated, very kind and sweet, and enjoying a high socioeconomic status, he was unable to express his feelings with his wife. After many sessions, he started a conversation with her about feelings and their sex life. He told her how unsatisfied he was. She didn't know how to answer or express herself in return.

"I feel horrible," he told me after.

They didn't have a good channel of communication, and it killed their love life. Richard showed what happens when the lack of communication and affection goes on too long.

Expression and Connection

How do you express yourself? Are you communicating well? Are you expressing your loving feelings? In what way? How do you relate your communication style to your culture or environment? How do you interpret your partner's loving expressions?

Pure Western culture, which most of us partake in, has two major components shaping it: materialism and individualism, which according to recent studies, are detrimental to health and well-being. Materialism places a high value on money and possessions rather than people. Materialism, according to Richard Eckersley from the National Centre for Epidemiology and Population Health of The Australian National University, "isn't associated with happiness but rather leads to anxiety, depression, anger, isolation, and alienation. The more materialistic we are, the poorer our quality of life."

Individualism places the individual at the center, celebrating personal freedom, independence, and choice, but according to Eckersley, it "has been taken too far or is misinterpreted." Eckersley explains that individualization has transformed identity into tasks, replacing our free will with obligation. There are so many people programmed to meet certain social standards that they feel obliged to self-determination. The result is real slavery and according to Eckersley, "the individualized life is a fate, not a choice; we cannot choose not to play the game."

Is this what it means to be free and independent?

I believe all this materialism and individualism not only reduces social connection, but also leads to disconnection from our partners, leading to poor intimacy. People are isolated and wallowing in subjective loneliness. Loneliness among American adults has increased by 16% in the last decade, according to recent researches. People are alone even while in a relationship! Connectivity is crucial for lovemaking. Connectivity drives love. We saw this clearly through the three examples above.

In fact, there are enough indicators that this is a real problem in our current society: the high divorce rate, couples living as roommates, increased depression, anxiety, mental illness, drug and alcohol abuse, high stress even in young people, suicide, and even mass shootings. Eckersley points out that Western society is falling short of maximizing human well-being. A large study of Americans aged 25-74 found that only 17% of people were "flourishing"—that is, they were enjoying good mental health—not only the absence of illness but, as most mental health professionals refer to it, "a syndrome of symptoms of positive feelings and positive functioning in life."

Why so few are "flourishing?" Because the lifestyle of Western society, where materialism and individualism prevail, is draining our mental health, happiness, and sex lives. In societies and contexts like this, how can we share love, express love, and make love?

This makes "the road" we take with our partner feel more like a "race" —go! go! go! —instead of like a "pleasant journey." To me, everything in America seems to be centered on work, success, achievement, money, who is better, and getting it done regardless of happiness and well-being. Is this how you want to "travel?" Can you make love in a "go! go! go!" way? I don't think so. Most likely, people are confusing having sex with lovemaking to the point of boredom and dissatisfaction. If this is your case, you are missing the best part of your relationship, the best part of your "journey." You will get bored, and you will probably stop expressing yourself. If you "travel" that way, you will be so focused "on the race" and your "goal"—with no time for conversations, romance, foreplays—that you will not be able to notice and enjoy your partner, feeling disconnected.

To be in an "unhealthy race" is a choice, not fate. Your other option is to enjoy a "pleasant journey" where lovemaking is possible. In a "pleasant journey," you can freely express yourself in words and actions, have effective communication, enjoy simple, silly conversation, and have intimacy, affection, pleasure, relaxation, smiles, laughter, music, and fun. It's never boring! Look at the Italians! They usually don't "race," they enjoy the "journey" —they make love more often.

Dr. Schwartz, mentioned in the previous chapters, indicates that "62% of couples in Italy have sex several times a week"—probably every day. In the U.S., we found an epidemic of "sexless couples," in which they have sex ten times per year or less! Dr. Schnarch, from Chapter 1, found that only 26% of couples have sex once a week—which is perceived as great and good enough for them. Also, it has been found that one in four Americans reports not having a single person to talk to about important issues. We need to improve!

More Love and Connection

A quote that I like from The Nap Ministry—found on Instagram @thenapministry—says: "you are exhausted physically and spiritually because the pace created by this system is for machines and not a magical and divine human being. You are enough. Rest." Yes, we need a break and rest to *make love 365 times a year*...

Ian Kerner, PhD, sex therapist and author of *She Come First* says, "when couples stop having sex, their relationships become vulnerable to anger, detachment, infidelity and, ultimately, divorce,"—beside all the mental and physical problems due to unhappiness, stress, and loneliness. Know that it is possible to *make love 365 times a year*! You could be American in your business life and Italian in your love life! Consciously choose to "perform" at work but be able to turn that off when you return home. Take time to find pleasure in the small things, express yourself, and leave your American work life behind you when you are with your partner. This is important, particularly for your health and the health of your relationship.

My vision is that more individuals and couples choose "a pleasant journey." Society itself could change in America if more people could be more aware of "the race," what it is, and the damage it causes, and instead, choose to enjoy small pleasure and make more love. This is the only way I see that we, as a society, can improve our own mental and physical health to heal our relationships—the foundation for functional families.

Indulge in your partner! Find pleasure in one another and make time for expressing your feelings. You need to be able to communicate with them to create a fulfilling love life. Expression is not only about verbally communicating your thoughts and ideas, talking, or having conversations; it is also about feelings, desires, and affection, non-verbal communication, facial expressions, gestures, movements, actions, inactions, unconscious truths, clothing, connection, and even smells!

Good communication skills are essential if you want to *make love 365 times a year...*

Communication

Communication is essential to organize, build, and maintain any relationship. Communication itself is the action of sending and receiving information. It is the primary way to select, to detect, to approach, to understand, to agree, and to consent. Healthy sexual expressions can't be accomplished without consent, which requires good communication—a unique and indispensable, universal tool to live with and share.

Connecting as a couple and staying connected through time is one of the most valuable tasks in any relationship; I would say it is one of the biggest challenges for couples. And you need great communication skills to accomplish that. Therefore, my Sex Secret #4 is expression, without which we cannot enjoy healthy and fulfilling relationships. We absolutely need proactive communication skills to find success as couples.

I find it interesting that one of the many steps inherent to all communication styles is motivation, a reason to talk. Basically, you want to communicate when you have a reason to do so. Information needs to be shared with other humans, especially with your partner. What is then the reason to communicate with your partner? The reasoning behind communication is very important when deciding why you want to communicate, what you want to communicate, and how you should communicate. Connection is the key word for couples!

Well-known author, entrepreneur, philanthropist, and life coach Tony Robbins states: "People often confuse communication for talking or making conversation, and this is the root cause of why many of these same people are so unsuccessful in communicating with their partners. Communication in relationships, at its core, is about connecting and using your verbal, written, and physical skills to fulfill your partner's needs—not just making small talk." The ultimate reason you should communicate with your partner is to connect and sustain that connection throughout your life. You can connect to your partner on many levels. Lovemaking, in my opinion, is the deepest level of connection. But how do you get there? How do you go so deeply into each other's souls?

As Angela R. Wiley, PhD, associate professor of the University of Illinois, says, "communication is a tool for knowing or emotionally connecting with one another." In her study on communication skills for healthy relationships, it was found that a positive emotional connection includes "having a partner who really talks to you, is a good listener, is a good friend, likes and appreciates you as a person, and does his or her share to make the relationship work." Communication between intimate partners is more than words—it involves establishing an emotional connection. Connecting through verbal and non-verbal communication is the cornerstone of emotional intimacy. You can have communication without emotional intimacy, but you CANNOT have emotional intimacy without communication! And, without emotional intimacy, we can't deeply connect to our partners. Therefore, it is best to learn first how to communicate effectively on a basic level, and then explore deeper levels.

Let's understand a little bit about communication. Communication is like "the head" of your relationship. You cannot have a relationship that doesn't think. Right? That will be an irrational relationship! There are many channels of communication open to you: spoken, written, body language, even your other senses. Without communication, there is no meaning to your relationship. Your relationship might seem "pretty," but it is empty—remember from the last chapter that love without intimacy is an empty love—probably full of misunderstanding, wrong interpretations, poor understanding, and deception. You and your partner will live like strangers!

Remember our analogy of the GPS and your car. Communication is what makes sure you and your partner are in the "same car," on the same journey! You don't want to be on two different roads, going in two different directions. Then you're no longer connecting, as we saw in each of the case studies. Sean Horan, PhD, an associate Professor in Interpersonal Communication, believes that "relationships are an incredible amount of work, and much of that work involves communication." He has found that communication is related to satisfaction within a relationship, as well as the couple's commitment to one another. Satisfaction and commitment are related to relationship persistence over time. Therefore, you cannot enjoy a healthy and satisfactory relationship without communicating.

Jennifer Priem, PhD, an associate Professor in the Communication Department at Wake Forest University, places interpersonal communication as "essential to individual's health and well-being." She has explored how messages of emotional support from a romantic partner facilitate physiological stress recovery. Communication is the skill needed to understand and relate to your partner at all levels. Always remember that, successful relationships require work and effort. Some people have the fairy tale romance in their head—a perfect partner will simply appear, and the relationship will be effortless. But this is real life! We need to communicate with our partners, understand them, listen to them, and empathize with them for the rest of our lives.

I have found in my practice that, in general, women tend to be more aggressive when trying to communicate—meaning, they pressure more to talk or express themselves—while men tend to be more passive—meaning, they exhibit more withdrawal behaviors and keep themselves in silence. Some men are also very aggressive to the point of becoming violent, while their partners remain passive to the point of submission. In any case, an aggressive style (confrontational), or a passive style (submissive) are both highly ineffective, especially for couple relationships.

Ineffective communication, then, just exacerbates problems and leads to disconnection. Avoiding difficult topics only make things worse! The prolongation of sensitive conversations just undermines your love life, and leads to nothing good...

Assertive Communication

Something I have noticed in my practice is that most couples lack assertiveness. This is a skill that you must gain, cultivate, and develop through practice. No one is born assertive! Think back to Richard in Case #4.3. His conversation about wanting to end his marriage was a very difficult one. But by working on his communication skills, he was able to have a tough conversation positively. This will promote healthy relationships through assertive communication, avoiding aggressive and passive styles.

Think about being assertive in this way: which of the three faces below would make you feel closer, more positive, understood, and welcome?

```
Aggressive style:
*Violent
*Guilt
*Need to
compensate
```

```
                    Assertive style:
                    *Feels good
                    *No need to take
                    or compensate
```

```
Passive style:
*Submissive
*Resentful
*Need to be
compensated
```

Assertiveness

Now, would you like your partner to be assertive when talking to you and have a pleasant face? Probably, yes! Then, do the same yourself! Smile and practice an assertive style when talking to your loved ones, to master it, regardless of the situation, so that you will feel closer, positive, understood, and welcome, and so will your partner. Aggressive and passive styles are very unproductive and lead to frustration. Assertiveness is the answer to a more productive, constructive, and proactive communication style to keep yourself connected while overcoming problems and understanding your differences.

Remember, good feelings are crucial to make love. Keep them positive and avoid resentment at all cost!

I recommend Judy Murphy's Book *Assertiveness: How to Stand Up for Yourself and Still Win the Respect of Others* which says assertiveness is "a style of communication that empowers its users. It's beyond being aggressive or passive but empowering yourself." The more you train yourself in assertive communication skills, the better your relationship with others will be, especially with your partner. Couples having chronic communication problems—either negative, reserved, withdrawn or violent—are couples that haven't been trained in assertive communication. Those couples suffer from lack of intimacy, dissatisfaction, disinterest on each other, and are probably experiencing the "Coolidge effect"—losing interest towards sex.

Research done by Claudia Sanchez Bravo and Alejandra Watty, published in the Journal of Sex & Marital Therapy in 2017, found that "one factor leading to marital dissatisfaction is communication, both the inability to communicate in certain areas and the way in which communication is made. Problems are aggravated by a lack of or ineffective communication. A couple with marital dissatisfaction is at greater risk for family violence, alcoholism, and drug abuse, which impacts their relationship, relationship with children, and work satisfaction." How your partner interprets what you say is an essential piece of your conversations. So, make sure he or she understood your message by asking them to repeat what you have said—that is paraphrasing.

Assertive communication has three parts: decision, sharing, and interpretation of the message. First, you decide what you want to share. You then impart the knowledge to your partner. But most importantly, is the interpretation of the message. Remember, the interpretation might be something different than what you believe your message said. Make sure that your message is clear, well elaborated and precise.

New Zealand communication expert Louise Shanly states that "communication is a two-way process of reaching mutual understanding in which participants not only exchange (encode-decode) information, news, ideas, and feelings but also create and share meaning. In general, communication is a means of connecting people or places." I like this definition in the way that communication is about understanding, meaning, and connection, especially if you want to build intimacy.

Brian Higginbotham, PhD, associate professor and extension specialist of Utah State University, suggests that "media usage at home should be limited, especially during quality time with one's partner. One example is limiting Internet usage. This is important for several reasons. It can interfere with quality couple and family interactions, and it can introduce a possible threat to relationship quality and fidelity."

Moreover, Wiley, mentioned before, unsurprisingly found that effective communication is critical for building and maintaining strong relationships. She proposed four simple tasks for successful and open verbal communication:

1. Keep it clear
2. Keep it soft
3. Keep it safe
4. Keep it positive

Non-Verbal Communication

World-renowned non-verbal communication expert, author of eleven books including Dangerous Personalities, and former FBI Special Agent Joe Navarro, defines non-verbal communication as "everything that communicates a message that is not a word." Professor, researcher, and expert on non-verbal communication Albert Mehrabian tells that verbal communication only makes up 7% of our communication, whereas 93% is non-verbal. The non-verbal component is made up of 55% body language, and 38% tone of voice. Therefore, the expressions of your body, the little movements and tiny gestures, should be highly important to truly understand each other.

Jeff Thompson, PhD, professor at New York University, crisis counselor, researcher, mediator, negotiator, and law enforcement detective, explains in Beyond Words that nonverbal communication is not only body language, it is also the environment, your clothing and appearance, touch, and your tone of voice. Thompson suggests that "when trying to understand others, a single gesture or comment does not necessarily mean something. Instead, these theories allow us to take note and observe more to get a better understanding of what is going on."

Pay attention to your partner's gestures and body language, not only their words. And more importantly, become aware of your own gestures, expressions, and movements. These could reveal a lot of you to your partner: unwanted feelings or unconscious desires that you do not need to share.

Micro-Expressions

Patryk & Kasia Wezowski, founders of the Center for Body Language, explain that we all learn from our parents or caregivers, negative facial expressions and micro-expressions that become unconscious to us, so we repeat them without realizing throughout our lives. They affirm that those micro-expressions are universal, so that anyone can decode them positively or negatively. They affirm that emotions lead to actions, and our reptilian brains control these micro-expressions, so these micro-expressions are really the most reliable signs of our emotions. The whole point is to learn that "micro-expressions are like road signs," according to Patryk & Kasia. So, you can manage your conversations by recognizing signs of disgust, disagreement, and happiness in order to spot, empower, and elicit positive emotions to sustain successful conversations.

So, observe more!

Navarro explains that non-verbal communication cannot be faked; remember that these are expressions that we aren't aware of most of the time. These expressions can be signs of comfort or discomfort that you must pay attention to. These non-verbal expressions can include touching one's face, covering one's eyes, biting one's lips, moving one's hands, neck movements, smiles, arm movements, etc. According to Navarro, "we are drawn to serenity," so be conscious of your micro-expressions and movements to make sure to attract your partner, not to push them away!

Navarro also emphasizes that "clothing does matter…at 6 months old, we already prefer beauty." How we look has an impact on our partners. Always make an effort to look your best; it is important to maintain the burning flame to make love. Be energetic, happy, and smile! These are the expressions of enthusiasm for your partner, that communicate without words that you care about them. Remember that non-verbal communication is more powerful than verbal, so show your appreciation and love, not only with words but also expressing them through your kind gestures—and, always smile!

Be aware that the brain is extremely sensitive to non-verbal expressions. The primitive or reptilian brain is the one in charge of picking and interpreting these expressions with no logical reasoning. Psychologist, author, and assistant clinical professor at the David Geffen School of Medicine, Dr. Stan Tatkin says, "threat detection is fundamentally a subcortical operation and may be understood as noncognitive…subcortical operation has a predilection for recognizing threatening facial expressions, vocal intonations, gestures, movements, and postures."

So usually, the primitive brain makes quick interpretations as threats. Our instinct to survive—the main function of the brain—is based on these threat detections, and any unconsciously learned micro-expression may be seen as a threat by others, "which may, in turn, lead either to violence or to systemic avoidance," according to Tatkin. Navarro also points out that "the minute you don't care, others won't care." Start by being the first in consciously modifying your verbal and non-verbal expressions, making communication effective with a purpose, so that you will find love, not war, in your relationship. Your partner, sooner or later, will follow you.

The process of consciously modifying your verbal and non-verbal expressions is not easy at all, but it is possible with some awareness and work. Mark Bowden, an expert in human behavior and body language, offers a great strategy for dealing with our non-verbal expressions. He suggests that you "be more unauthentic to each other the rest of your life because if you don't choose your behaviors beyond your natural instincts, for what you like and don't like, you will miss brilliant opportunities in your life." That suggestion makes a lot of sense to me, according to what we have learned about unconscious micro-expressions.

As Bowden says, "you have to choose your behaviors and expressions." Remember that when you are talking to your partner, your partner's primitive brain will automatically pick your non-verbal expressions without thinking, probably interpreting them as threats and sabotaging your good intentions. Therefore, by being "inauthentic," you are truly "authentic" since you are choosing your expressions consciously and not letting your unconscious behavior—learned in childhood—to control the present moment. You are authentic when you consciously decide to express what you are feeling now.

Please, be aware that there is something in our nature that will prevent us from being staying in love, connected over time. That is what Bowden fantastically explains as, "we all are designed by nature to be indifferent to each other," so we won't pay attention to people around us unless certain expressions trigger our reptile or primitive brain, placing the person in front of us, according to Bowden, into one of these three categories: "friend, enemy, or potential sexual partner." That categorization depends on expressions such as smiles, eye contact, maintenance of eye contact, hand movements, and other expressions.

How do you want your partner to categorize you? Do you see why a great and passionate relationship requires a lot of work and maintenance? Remember in Chapter 3, where I explain that for a couple to keep "the burning flame," they need to pay attention to each other and keep the good feelings? How can you do this if you are indifferent to your partner? Be aware of your expressions as well as your vocabulary—how you are expressing yourself—to *make love 365 times a year*!

Good communication skills—verbal and non-verbal—are a determining factor for your happiness in all aspects of your life, such as work, family, love, sex, friends, etc. Building up these abilities will help you across the board. Your assertive communication skills are suitable when building intimacy. You will need these skills throughout your entire life. Communication and intimacy are highly related, but not the same thing. You cannot build intimacy without communication. Intimacy is a deeper communicational level that you must build with your partner for a healthy relationship. As Tony Robbins says, "a couple can build intimacy by practicing effective communication in relationships."

Once you and your partner can hold constructive talks, you can be ready to enjoy true emotional and sexual intimacy—deeper levels of interaction—to *make love 365 times a year…*

Part II: Emotional Intimacy

Now we are entering into a deeper sphere most couples are afraid of: Emotional intimacy! We all need to build emotional intimacy in our relationships to establish a solid connection with our partner, and this requires time, perseverance, patience and effort, since it is not easy and involves discomfort and risks. People usually confuse intimacy with sex. Don't! Intimacy is NOT sex or about sex; it is about disclosing true feelings and emotions in a conscious, safe, and open way. It's about open communication! All couples communicate—poorly, aggressively, passively, assertively, non-verbally, verbally—and this may dictate how strong their emotional intimacy is.

There is a great way to think of intimacy—intimacy is: *into-me-see.* You are now looking "into" your partner's soul through their feelings, and they are looking into yours. Sexologist Dr. Kat Smith, an intimacy expert, says "intimacy is the foundation for relationships. It's about connection with your own emotions and with your partner's emotions—your needs, desires, and hopes." Intimacy is communication at a deeper level, of private and personal information where vulnerability and risks take place.

Recall that you can have communication without intimacy, but you CANNOT have intimacy without communication. Here you are expressing, sharing and disclosing your deepest thoughts, wishes, dislikes, likes, fears, and dreams. You are truly laying your soul bare while allowing your partner to "see" into you. A study done by Dr. Niveen Rizkalla found that 70% of couples consider themselves happy, but not intimate. These couples do not have a warm connection or truly know one another, probably because "intimacy forces you outside your comfort zone," as Rizkalla says.

There are three ingredients that Rizkalla proposes for creating emotional intimacy:

1. Exposure: talking about feelings, emotions, hopes, dreams, fears.
2. Responsiveness: the way you respond to one another with sensitivity and caring.
3. Capacity to be alone: you know yourself and can balance being alone and being together as a couple, alone, just the two of you.

Most couples avoid this level of intimacy. Most likely it is because they are scared to open themselves up to their partner—sometimes is risky. They fear rejection or being ignored, misunderstood, not appreciated, or manipulated. People worry their partners, the one person they should trust most in life, will make fun of or tease them. So instead they refuse to communicate. But the only way you can achieve emotional intimacy is through this sharing...

Remember, communication is like the "head" of your relationship. It is what makes you think and solve problems; it gives you the skills you need. Now intimacy is like the "heart," what makes you express your feelings. You need both to connect to your partner—but sometimes head and heart aren't in accord. Only when they are synchronized, can you feel secure, confident, certain, and committed. Only then can your decision-making be on track for you to have a healthier relationship. You need to develop intimacy just as much as communication skills.

As I mentioned before, intimacy is about disclosure. But disclosure of what? Self-disclosure of your present feelings and emotions, the disclosure of the real you in the present moment. Clinical psychologist, sex therapist, and author of *The Pleasure Zone*, Stella Resnick, PhD, wisely says that when we are trying to honestly disclose ourselves, we often think we are telling the truth, but this is only what we think is the truth—what it's in our head.

The truth is, according to Resnick, that "you may simply be repeating an old story you've been telling yourself for years…a reflection of something you believe and not something you feel, it's not a true reflection of the real you. Self-revelation involves just being with another person and discovering your feelings in the moment." To disclose yourself to your partner, you need to know your feelings first. You need to feel! And to feel, you need to be present! This is the reason we discussed finding yourself first in previous chapters. How can you share yourself if you don't know yourself? Clinical psychologist Dr. Sue Johnson says, "knowing yourself increases intimacy. To know your hopes, dreams, thoughts, ambitions and to tell your partner."

Schnarch, mentioned before, says that "intimacy is often misunderstood as necessarily involving acceptance, reciprocity, and validation from one's partner… Intimacy is not the same as closeness, bonding, or care-taking. It is an "I-Thou" experience. It involves the inherent awareness that you are separate from your partner." know yourself and then show yourself to your partner. Validate your partner when they do the same for you! Do not try to change them! You don't even have to agree with them, but instead recognize, accept, and understand your partner—see-into-him or her.

Resnick in *The Heart of Desire*, clarifies that "what's important is not just how well we communicate verbally but also what two bodies are saying to each other when they're together, whether the message is mentally registered or not." Remember the non-verbal communication and your micro-expressions. Along the way, you will start believing your long-term partner already understands you. Instead of assuming you are in accord, talk to one another all the time, and make sure always to express your feelings to keep yourselves connected. As Resnick says, "in a loving relationship, both partners can become better acquainted with their own true selves, along with the true self of the other…describing your experience without trying to explain or justify it."

True emotional intimacy and connection is the most precious gift you can give to each other. That intimate connection will allow you to have the capacity to, not only regulate your own self in times of adversity, but also to learn how your partner regulates themselves. In fact, Tatkin recommends that you and your partner "must become expert on each other and know what to do in any cases of distress. Both are in each other's care, and not simply their own…in a cross-care, mutual regulation…in a good co-regulatory team." I believe so, too: you and your partner are one team, so work and help each other as "a team" to regulate yourselves, grow, and *make love 365 times a year.*

Remember from Chapter 2 the importance of time management. Time is fundamental to your love life. Tatkin emphasizes that "time is essential for error correction and repair, to fine-tune meanings and to engage in the back and forth of error correction needed for successful verbal communication." So, placing your partner as a priority in your life and making the time to communicate and build emotional intimacy, is the path to a satisfying relationship.

But be careful of building intimacy with the wrong person! Especially on the Internet, it can be easy to open yourself up and share your deepest thoughts and fears, because you really are not with the other person. If they judge you, it is less painful than if your partner judges you. Their rejection doesn't have the same sting. Like we discussed in Chapter 3, this feeling of anonymity can lead to cheating on your partner. Likewise, some people may put this weight on their friends, parents, or even their children. The emotional heaviness inside of you should go to your partner!

The process will be much easier, if you do it with understanding and affection, making your experience more comfortable and rewarding.

Affection and Touching: Key Elements for Emotional Intimacy

Do you remember the impact that culture plays on your love life? Pay attention to how unimportant affection is in Western cultures, especially touch. How we communicate with one another is very important—especially with our partner. It is through communication that we show our affection for one another. When we first think of communication, most people think of talking. But touch is just as important, if not more important, than our words, especially in romantic relationships.

It is through a combination of talking and touch that we show our affection for our partner, the most important and powerful expression that, according to Resnick, is *healing*. She affirms that "loving touch is healing. Touch that senses the other is a silent way of speaking and listening to each other." Without affection, you cannot be in a healthy romantic relationship. Without it, you don't have a partner, just a roommate. When there is no affection, there is no connection. Your relationship is platonic, not tender. You might be able to talk well, but without affection, and the touch that goes with it, you aren't deeply connecting.

So, let's learn more about affection! The basic definition of affection says it is "a feeling of liking and caring for someone or something, a tender attachment, fondness." More importantly, it is also "a physical way of showing just how much you love someone. It is a fondness that consumes you, wanting to touch, tickle, kiss, hug, or hold." Affection is the expression of your positive feelings. It is a very powerful way of communicating. Affection CANNOT be missing if you are planning on *making love 365 times a year.* Some people I talk to worry because they have never seen affection before. Their parents didn't express it, so they feel lost. But affection can be learned! Think of it like this—if your parents were poor when you were young, you were poor too, right? But as an adult, you don't have to remain poor anymore if you decide so; it's up to you now! This applies to everything. You can make changes to your own life now.

Sociologist and psychologist Dr. Mark Knapp, tells us that "tacit communication is the most basic, or primitive form of communication." It's important because affection is the verbal and physical expression of your love. You cannot make love without love and affection. Constant affection enhances your physiological functioning. Ongoing displays of affection "feed" your relationship and keep it strong! Sadly, a lack of affection is the number one reason that couples in America seek therapy, according to recent studies.

Touching

Communication professor Sean M. Horan, PhD, found that "the frequency with which you expressed affection to, and received affection from a partner was directly related to your commitment and satisfaction—and research documents that satisfaction and commitment are important, as they predict relational persistence over a 15-year period." Broken down, that means that couples that showed more affection were more likely to stay together. The amount of affection received from your partner was the strongest indicator of satisfaction. The amount of affection expressed to your partner was the strongest indicator of commitment.

And by far, the best way to express affection is through touching! There have been so many studies over the years showing how important touch is to the human psyche. A famous study in the 1990s looked at Romanian orphans over their childhood and early life. These children received little to no touch from any parental figures, and later in life expressed significant emotional, psychological, and physical health problems, all from a lack of touch in their childhood.

Dr. Sue Carter, neurobiologist and the Director of the Kinsey Institute, states that "without loving relationships or in isolation, humans fail to flourish, even if all of their other basic needs are met. They need a sense of safety, which in turn allows social cognition, social bonding, social support, growth, and restoration." So, touching is love and love is growth! It creates increased levels of oxytocin, which make your body feel good and connected to your loved one. We all need this oxytocin to thrive.

A positive look at the importance of touch is a study done on the NBA by Michael W. Kraus, Cassy Huang, and Dacher Keltner in the peer-reviewed journal Emotion. They tracked the amount of touching a team does and looked for any correlation with how that team might play. The players who touched their teammates more, through high fives, fist bumps, or hugs, had higher win scores, defined as "a performance measure," and they enjoyed significantly superior team performance that those that touch less. Pedro and I are fan of the Barcelona soccer team. I've noticed that when they score a goal, it's amazing how they hug, touch each other, express affection, and celebrate. I haven't seen a more powerful friendship on a field! Barcelona is an affective, highly effective, winning, strong and powerful team! One more proof of the benefits of affection and touch.

Now, if that happens to sports teams, imagine how it can work for your own team: you and your partner! You two are the most important team there is. So why aren't you touching more? If you want to succeed and have a happy, fulfilling and satisfying relationship, you must touch more! No excuses! Touch is free, safe, easy, and fun. If you don't know how, learn! It's not about sex, it's about affection…

Learning to Touch

Staying together for years isn't a good measure of success and relationship satisfaction. I have seen couples who have been together for 35 years or more and can't stand to touch one another. What a neglectful kind of love! This is not a success! A fulfilling relationship is one where you are happy, satisfied, and longing to stay. Affection is key!

Jane Anderson, in *The Power of Touch*, beautifully says that "the hand has the ability to be an extension of the heart to give and to receive. Touch can decrease violence and depression and increase immunity and trust bounds. The only sense we cannot live without is touch. Touch is the mother of all senses. Our first language! Touch is powerful communication tool." Therefore, if you truly want trust and happiness in your relationship, then touch more and ask for more!

Moreover, eye contact is also highly important when expressing yourself and being affectionate. Resnick explains that "two loving people can silently transmit information back and forth through eye contact as well as touch that can adjust each other's heart rate, hormone levels, disease fighting blood cells, and more. This is called entrainment or neural synchrony."

Make touching and affection love habits. Talk and touch from the very beginning of the day. Remember my fun and hot exercise that I suggested in Chapter 2—Pretzel Time—to connect and release the amazing attachment hormones. Also, my earlier suggestion of the four kisses—one when you wake up, one when you leave for work, one when you return home, and one at night. French kiss more and hug your partner more...with no sexual expectations. These are powerful love habits to build and sustain a daily connection through touching.

Touch even when you do not have to. Congratulate each other, even if it's something small. Kiss unexpectedly and without reason. In a study done by Kory Floyd, it was found that kissing can lower cholesterol levels, decrease stress, and increase relationship satisfaction. Communicating our positive feelings for each other through words and touch can also lower blood pressure and lead to a stronger immune system. And these benefits happen when affection is expressed, not merely felt. In fact, you can get a health boost from expressing affection even if the receiver doesn't reciprocate! According to Floyd, "a hug may not change anything about what's going bad in your day, but it can change how you feel in that moment. It feels like all of your stress is just melting away."

In my practice, I encourage couples to have, what I call, "an affection week" for them getting used to giving and receiving tons of affection daily. It's a week where you consciously and massively give and receive all kinds of affection in different ways: compliments, kissing, hugging, writing notes, and snuggling, all in a non-sexual way. Associating sex with affection is very common and may lead to disconnection. Couples usually only touch affectionately when they are going to have sex. This can be a major problem! When this happens, eventually, you will begin to correlate affection with sex, which is wrong! If you don't feel like having sex at that moment, then you're also giving up affection.

Don't starve emotionally! If you associate giving affection with sex, then you will not have pure affection. No sex = no affection; no affection = no sex—too bad for your relationship. Sex and affection are different expressions; they can work nicely together but need to be expressed independently. I encourage couples to reflect on this and learn to experience sex and affection in a separate way to distinguish each feeling. For example, to be very affectionate and tender with no sexual intentions. Women have learned to express affection, love, and intimacy easily to get closer to their partners. There is nothing wrong with that, but I encourage them to express sexual desires explicitly.

On the other hand, men have learned to express themselves sexually, in many cases, inhibiting feelings. I encourage them to express love and emotions explicitly, as well. The desire for sex and affection are healthy expressions that should be part of a love equation. Both expressions are important, and both can be expressed by men and women. Just learn and practice!

Then you can be affectionate without worrying if you will have sex or not. And, if you learn to make love and integrate it as part of your daily routine, you will have less to worry about. Just experience the pure pleasure of touch; your relationship can survive even when you aren't having sex for any reason. Affection doesn't have to die because sex does. Once you have uncoupled sex and affection, you can become more erotic.

Part III: Sexual Intimacy

Now we are entering in an even deeper sphere, that most couples crave: sexual intimacy! As Dr. Schwartz says, "sex is a strong expression of a deep emotional connection between two people." Now sexual intimacy is: Into-me-see *and feel*—inside of me, feeling me. Emotional intimacy, as we have seen, involves both emotional and physical interactions with total closeness and openness, but without sexual interactions. When all the elements of emotional intimacy are combined, and the sexual component is added, the mixture is explosive, unique, and fascinating! It is the emergence of sexual intimacy, which leads to a unique and exclusive connection.

Sexual intimacy is the *expression* of your sexual being that includes your sexual desires, sexual fantasies, wants, uncertainties, and even fears about sex. This intimacy is about knowing your partner sexually, opening to your partner to explore sexual feelings—yours and your partner's—and completely freeing sexually in each other presence—a state that is often reserved for just one person in the whole world. Sexual intimacy is the physical embodiment of emotional intimacy. I believe deep penetration takes place here, without intercourse, when genuine expressions of pleasure touch your soul…

In this level, you don't just take your hearts out, but your clothes off, along with your social masks, defense mechanisms, fears, doubts, and insecurities. This intimate space is created for exploring who you and your partner really are, where shared sexualities take place and are expressed. There is no other space like this! It's your heaven on Earth! Enter the realm of pleasure and sensations where freedom—and nothing else—should reign. You will feel each other as never before, each time you make love, each time you kiss...so, surrender and JUST FEEL! This is the perfect "space" that will allow you to *make love 365 times a year* and remain deeply connected...

While emotional intimacy is more verbal than physical, sexual intimacy is more physical than verbal—skins are talking. You should now feel safe and secure due to the creation of trust. Once you are fearless, available, and secure, you must build and hold up your sex life with open hearts, open minds, open bodies, and open souls. You should now sexually self-disclose and disrobe with your partner. Nothing is hidden; your true identities are bare. Your sexuality is exposed to your partner. I am not talking about sex; it is much more than that. Lovemaking is not necessarily an expression of sexual desires; it is an expression of your love for each other...to deeply hold each other...

Please be aware that lovemaking is different than just having sex, as we discussed in Chapter 3. Lovemaking should be the essence of your sex life. I am talking about the deep bonding of two bodies, including bare genitals. Therapist, intimacy and relationship coach, and clinical supervisor Amy Color indicates that "intimacy and connection can't just be talked about, they need to be experienced." Both expressions and actions are equally important to your sex life and sexual intimacy. The whole experience—words and actions—is sexual intimacy. But how to experience love and connection on a deeper level?

One powerful way to experience a deeper level of connection is through your senses. You both need to:

- ▶ Taste—lick, bite, suck, kiss a lot
- ▶ Smell—smell the odors of each other, the environment (be sure it's pleasant—no kid smells!)
- ▶ Sight—see each other naked, look at each other eye-to-eye for long periods, observe micro-expressions.
- ▶ Touch—caressing, touching, feeling, exploring textures and pressures
- ▶ Hear—hear the most primitive expressions, dirty language, sighs of pleasure. As it is said, "the clitoris is in the ears of women."

Of all these sensory scans, smelling is the most important, which I will discuss in Chapter 6. Hearing is also very significant, since while in your private space, you hear each other's primitive and unique expressions—little sounds of pleasure, moans, exclamations, and sighs. You make love in your own language... These short, unsophisticated, natural, spontaneous noises show that you feel free with one another. Share them with your lover!

All your senses are vital to lovemaking...

Clinical psychologist and professor Dr. Sue Johnson suggested that "making love is the ultimate moment of communal in a relationship. The biggest factor in the quality of your sexual relationship is the safety of your emotional connection with the person you are making love with. We are bonding animals first and foremost. We need that emotional connection to feel safe in our own skin. Which is even more powerful than lust."

An intimate space like this, safe enough to freely experience deep pleasure, is truly powerful as well as healthy because:

1. Reduces fear in the brain
2. Solidifies trust
3. Provides feelings of safety
4. Lowers defense mechanisms
5. Deeply connects you to your partner
6. Increases your desire to be together and make love over and over!
7. Increases trust as love grows stronger...

And, the best and easy way to induce this fantastic cascade is by doing Pretzel Time as soon as you wake up—and why not lovemaking? What a great, easy, and fun way to *make love 365 times a year*! I can reassure you that you will love to make love every day...

Finding Sexual Intimacy

The more you trust, the less afraid you are, and more you want to make love. Robert Taibbi, a clinical social worker, explains that "exposing our intimate thoughts and wishes can make us feel self-critical, small, or unsafe. We fear judgement or rejection."

Therefore, it is imperative to make an effort to consciously build trust before having difficult conversations about sex. Once you have a secure space where you can trust and feel safe, you will have the sexual intimacy you both need to be able to easily express your sexual concerns, likes, dislikes, fantasies, desires, and fears. In no time you may feel naturally aroused when you interact intimately, by getting used to and being positively conditioned to feel, see, and smell each other. Your brain knows the marvelous things that await you... Then, you will have created love habits that will allow you to enjoy your sexuality–no pills needed!

In fact, you will be drawn by your partner's smells, expressions, and petting, making you ready for lovemaking—where all fears are gone. LOVEX—from Chapter 3—is fundamental for lovemaking, and lovemaking is the perfect space to experience LOVEX in all its glory! Your bodies are now the ones "conversing..." See? It is possible to *make love 365 times a year*; you must act and set the space for it to occur. Believe is healthy for you, for your partner, and for your relationship, and behave in ways to fulfill such a wonderful challenge.

According to Dr. Johnson, "when we feel securely connected to somebody, we can be open to new ideas, courteous, explore, and take risks. This is especially true for women. Women need to talk and check out the relationship before they can let themselves go and descend into arousal. Talking is a key part of foreplay (for women) …how you connect emotionally is how you can connect sexually. Being connected to your partner opens you up for erotic play."

If you are not safe, or your partner doesn't feel safe, then you cannot "play." Think about a small child—a securely, well-adapted, attached child—can experience their world free of their mother. He/she knows the mother won't disappear, and while he/she may check in from time to time, he/she has the confidence to explore the world on his/her own. It is kind of the same here. Within your relationship, you need to feel safe to explore yourself, your partner, your fantasies. But again, and again, you must feel safe first in order to "playing" with your partner in bed.

Dr. Mike Anderson, an expert in communication, says, "sex is top of the list of taboo topics in relationships. Sexual fantasies are top of the top of taboo subjects." Anderson ran experiments to see how sexual fantasies affect relationships and found that intimate couples who disclose sexual fantasies have higher sexual satisfaction and relationship satisfaction. By broaching this "taboo" subject, we actually made our relationship stronger!

Four benefits have been found from talking about sexual fantasies:

1. Couples can decide to act out fantasies
2. Sex life improvement

3. The establishment of a deeper bond
4. Opens communication even more

Anderson proposed three levels of fantasies. We all fall into one of these categories, so what are yours? Let's see them:

Level 1: Detailed and elaborate fantasy: In your fantasy, there is a storyline, characters, and setting, with precise details.
Level 2: Less elaborate but still creative fantasy: Your fantasy maybe is a simple storyline with some characters and few or no details.
Level 3: Very simple fantasy: Your fantasy is just thoughts and passing ideas; there is no storyline and no specific characters.

Interestingly, Anderson found that the lowest level of sexual satisfaction is found among those with Level 1 fantasies, because there is a tendency not to share them. In other words, they are intricate, thought-out fantasies their partner doesn't know about. They are specific and descriptive, but not shareable, because of the partner's reaction. Now you are no longer communicating; you have fears. Anderson concluded: "It is very important to have sexual fantasies and to share them with your partner to have a better sex life. And establish deeper connection and bonds, and to have a deeper communication." And this deeper communication is sexual intimacy.

If you have Level 1 fantasy (which is great), it is likely you will keep your fantasy hidden for fear of rejection. When in fear, we can't disclose our hidden self to one another. Dr. Ellis expressed that "American boys and girls, and later American men and women, believe sex is good and bad. Tasty and nasty. They are in a word conflicted. Conflict means indecision and doubt, which means fear… As we inhabit and deaden our tender reactions, we also block some of our deepest sexual reactions. To the extent that we have little love, we tend to have more fear, including sex fear." This fear Dr. Ellis referred to is exactly what will keep you from consistent lovemaking…

As Amy Color says, "without intimacy people feel lonely, isolated, and shame. It doesn't matter if you have sex every day. What is missing is intimacy. It's the loss of intimacy that causes partners to become roommates. That lack of intimacy is the most common reason for relationship break downs." As I explained in Chapter 3, intimacy is necessary to lovemaking. Remember that one of the components of LOVEX, according to my model, is intimacy—emotional and sexual. We need LOVEX to make love!

When, Where, and How to Talk About Sex

Now the typical questions: when, where, and how to talk about sex? First, get over your fear and doubts by facing "the elephant in the room." Remember that is crucial that you and your partner generate a secure space to hold conversations about sex. That is one of the reasons you should have this space, to freely talk about private matters, such as sex and sexuality.

As you feel more comfortable taking about your dreams, feelings, and fantasies, make sure you start incorporating conversations about sex. Little by little, you will be desensitized; that is, you will become uninhibited little by little so that, in no time, you will be taking about sex regularly, as a normal topic in your conversations. Don't be afraid to talk about your sexual needs and desires; incorporate them whenever it is appropriate.

Consciously setting space to talk about sex is fundamental to keep your sex life alive and vice versa. It is a task you and your partner must accomplish to prevent frustration and misunderstandings in the bedroom. The truth is that most couples do not talk openly and maturely about their sexual needs, and some don't talk about it at all. Conversations about sex are usually taken for granted, and that is what brings problems, disconnection, and discomfort. In fact, bad and boring sex could come from this lack of expression of sexual needs and tastes—lack of communication and intimacy.

Since the topic is usually avoided, neglected, or is postponed, you need to set up a time and place to talk exclusively about sex. Whatever works for you and your partner is good, as long as you can openly express your sexual concerns and thoughts. Just like Robert did in Case #4.3—you may want to plan for this task ahead of time.

Here are seven simple steps to follow when having conversations about sex, so that you will feel comfortable and not awkward:

1. Talk about talking! If you find yourself feeling awkward about sex talks, then set up a conversation to agree to set up another conversation to talk about sex!
2. Decide what you want to say in 3 or 4 simple concrete points. Elaborate on your concerns, opinions, suggestions, or point of view before the

conversation. Be very specific and name body parts and sexual activities by their names. Your genitals are part of your body, and they are as normal and important as any other body part.

3. Set up a good time and place for BOTH of you, making sure it is a relaxing setting where you won't have discomfort, distractions or interruptions.

4. Follow the rule "I"—start sentences with "I" and avoid starting with "you." It is about your feelings, desires, fantasies, thoughts, suggestions, questions, or needs, not about your partner's.

5. Feel comfortable when expressing your sexual self; there is nothing wrong or bad about sexual thoughts. Inhale, exhale, and relax, then FOCUS on the points you already elaborated on. Help your partner feel comfortable and relaxed, as well. Be kind, gentle, empathic, respectful and compassionate. Compassion and empathy are essential for deep connection.

6. Ask your partner to paraphrase your words and vice versa to make sure everything is understood. Make error corrections as needed by clarifying misunderstandings without being defensive, upset, or frustrated. That is why you are talking!

7. Talk about talking more! Generate options and agree on the ones both of you feel good about. Go ahead and make it happen! Enjoy your talk, planning, and materializing your ideas. Plan to follow up after your conversation. Make it fun!

Next, touch each other with no expectations. Break the habit of affection=sex! Just express your love with your hands, heart, and body. You've already used your words to express your love; now use touch. Try some of these:

▶ Touch each other's face while gazing into each other's eyes.
▶ Practice the kissing. Go from small kisses and bites to French kissing. Give a deep, three-minute kiss while hugging.
▶ Touch every part of each other's bodies except the genitals. Enjoy and get to know each other's bodies.
▶ Touch with intention and attention, then explore each other's genitals with appreciation, if desired to orgasm.

Try for a sublime experience with no expectations and only the intention of connection. Never shut one another down, no matter what the other wants to try.

This is not about penis-in-vagina sex; it's about building your sexual connection as a romantic couple. The point is that you are two individuals joining your hearts, feelings, and bodies into a single sublime expression of love. You are making love!

Know that during this experience, unhappy feelings and painful memories can be triggered because of past trauma. This is, then, the place to overcome misery together, with your safe and trusted partner. You cannot fully experience sexual pleasure with unresolved past trauma. Lovemaking can become a healing power to rescue you from the past and bring you to the present for a wonderful future together... It's about the two of you naked, not only your bodies but your souls...

Remember that familiarity is what makes lust get lost! And you need some lust for a balanced love life full of passion and intimacy—LOVEX. If lust gets lost, it will be hard to make love in a fun way. The best relationships understand that there are two people in a relationship. The love, caring, and intimacy between these people still allow space for them to be their own people, with their own desires, dreams, and fears. Sexual intimacy is not about having the same sexual desires, dreams, sexual frequencies, and fears, but is about recognizing and owning your feelings and respecting your partner's. Don't lose yourself! Find and know who you are, and your partner as well, by expressing yourselves.

Part IV: Building Intimacy—The Three-Floor House

Based on Nina's E. *Six-Dimensional Model of Marital Communication*, 1991, —1. Feelings, emotions, and dislikes. 2. Extended Family, 3. Sexuality, 4. Marital relationship. 5. Work. 6. Children—I propose a Three-Dimensional Model regarding levels of interaction in marital/romantic committed relationships for increasing intimacy. I have organized Nina's six dimensions into three categories or "levels of interaction," which I have called: *The Three-Floor House: Heinz Three-Dimensional Levels of Interaction*, to graphically differentiate and organize the types of communication and interactions within healthy committed relationships, as well as how to build emotional and sexual intimacy.

To explain my model, I have used the analogy of a pyramid house with three floors to illustrate and describe these three levels of interaction within—healthy—committed relationships. I propose my model in a straightforward, graphic, and organized way so that everyone can understand what it means to build up a healthy relationship, with room for intimacy. So, think of a house with three stories in a pyramid shape. The bottom floor supports the second floor, and the second floor supports the third floor. In that same way, these three dimensions support one another. You cannot hop magically to the third floor without having the two other solid floors beneath you.

According to the *Three-Floor-House: Heinz Three-Dimensional Levels of Interaction*, the three levels of interactions are:

Level 1 (1st Floor): Environmental Level: Interaction with the environment—Nina's 2. Extended Family. 5. Work. 6. Children. This Level or "Floor" is all about family, friends, work, careers, household, children, money, and you and your partner as individuals with individual goals. This Level is where interaction with your environment occurs; that is, it includes both you and your environment. The environmental life level of interaction is your foundation as a structure. It contains all the aspects concerning your family, including inside factors such as children, extended family living with you, house chores, pets, money management, debts, the to-do list, duties, and the whole functioning of your home.

This level also includes outside factors such as work, education, the Internet and the media, religion, politics, family businesses, extended families not living with you, your community, neighbors, friends, etc. A relationship starts with two people, so everything starts here: you and your partners as two separated individuals with your own unique set of problems, virtues, possibilities, dreams, and goals. Your individual spaces lie at this level. You are two people with different projects, willing to give, receive, and share whatever you have.

Communication, conversations, and dialog with your partner are about your environment and your individual projects. In Level 1, "you are a family," which includes all the people around you who have or could have something to do with you and your family in any way. Each member of the family has a personal project and a unique life to be respected and appreciated. In relation to the Sternberg Theory of Love—mentioned in Chapter 3—Level 1, or "1st Floor," would be the Commitment Level.

Level 2 (2nd Floor): Relational Level: Interaction as "a couple" within the relationship per se—Nina's 1. Feelings, emotions, and dislikes. 4. Marital relationship. This Level or "Floor" is more about feelings, emotions, conversations between the two of you, discussions about likes and dislikes, and activities as a couple. This level is where interactions with your partner "as a couple" occur. The couple life level is the foundation of your love life. Here your common projects, as a couple, lie, and here is where you need to feed, maintain, regain, and rebuild your connection as a team couple. It is where you become "one" by having the same project in common.

This level, or "Floor," is where emotional intimacy takes place, between you and your partner. The "us with clothes." Every aspect that only concerns the two of you. This level includes communication of feelings, emotions, ideas, plans, thoughts, personal and couples' goals, agreements and disagreements, recreational activities as a couple, romance and romantic activities, dates, love and affection, seduction, and the most important aspect: emotional intimacy, where the deepest connection begins to evolve. Affection is essential at this level and quality time with your partner is imperative! In Level 2, "you are a couple," which only admits you and your partner, or primary partner. Here the two of you become one in intentions, projects, and desires. In relation to the Sternberg Theory of Love, Level 2—2nd Floor— would be the Intimacy Level.

Level 3 (3rd Floor): Sexual Level: Interactions as sexual partners, "lovers"—Nina's 3. Sexuality. This level is where lovemaking and sexual interaction occur, where sexuality evolves. Your sexual level of interaction is the foundation for lovemaking. This level is where sexual intimacy takes place—the two of you as one; where penetration of the soul occurs, not only that of the body. The "us with no clothes." This level is the perfect space to create LOVEX—see Chapter 3. Here is where your two bodies become one when *making love 365 times a year.*

This level of interaction goes far beyond orgasms and sexual activities; it is about transcendent connection, sexual intimacy, freedom, exploration, and spirituality—the top of the cake! A unique, sacred, secret, and special place. Sexualities, sexual mindsets and expressions, fantasies, satisfaction and sexual pleasures are exposed to be lived fully. This space is the most intimate space of all, there is no place like this. The decision to include others in this level is totally up to you, as long as it is consensual.

Conversation and interactions at this level are more sensual and sexual, inclined towards sexual expressions. It is the space where you experience total permission to be yourselves. In Level 3 "you are lovers," which allows no expectations, no masks, no clothes, no appearances, no rules, no restrictions, no chores, no duties, no obligations: only free, non-judgmental, consensual, and pleasurable activities. Only the two of you, feeling one another, exploring, and becoming emotional and sexually happy. This level is the deepest level of connection. This "floor" —the 3rd Floor or Level 3—should become "your heaven on Earth!" It's for me, and my wish is that it's for you too… In relation to the Sternberg Theory of Love, Level 3— 3rd Floor—would be the Passion Level.

The Three-Floor House

Let's look at the "Three-Floor House" model to illustrate how a healthy couple interrelates on each level—according to my model—and thus, creating the spaces for emotional and sexual intimacy. Let's explore how you could adapt this model to build and keep your relationship healthy and passionate throughout the years, to *make love 365 times a year.*

I have found in my practice that dysfunctional and unhappy couples stop interacting as "a couple," that is, they only interact as "a family." These couples only experience interactions in Level 1 (on the 1st Floor) and very little or nothing at Levels 2 and 3—giving up their "2nd and 3rd Floors." Frequently, these couples do not have joint projects, communicate poorly, and are disconnected. Usually, they only operate as good friends, roommates, parents, or co-workers. If that's what you want, that's fine, but you're missing a large part of what it means to be in a complete, passionate relationship.

Remember from Chapter 3 that, having sex is not the same as making love. According to this model, the sexual level of interaction, Level 3, is about sexual intimacy, which is beyond "having sex." It is a space for sexual connection, pleasure, and satisfaction. Do you want to *make love 365 times a year*? So, let's strengthen your 1st and 2nd Floors" first and then build a solid 3rd Floor to make love!

Let's see the Three-Floor House: Heinz Three-Dimensional Levels of Interaction:

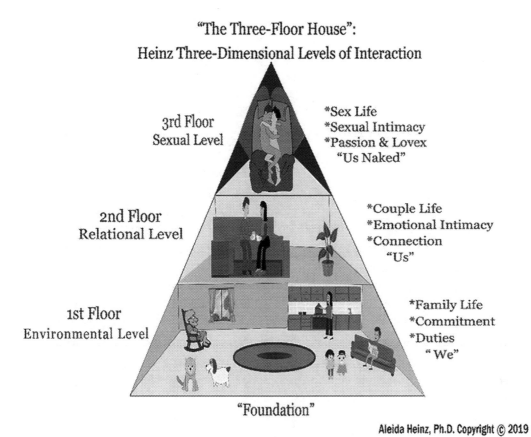

The Three-Floor House Model

Building Your Three-Floor House

The "1st Floor" is your day to day stuff you need to do to keep your lives going. It is a vast, spacious "floor;" the foundation of your "house." Unfortunately, most couples in long-term relationships prioritize this "floor" and underestimate the other two. You can easily get stuck here! Talking about nothing but work, chores, whose turn it is to get the children—if you have—what your uncle or a friend said today, the weather, etc. You may be distracted by different things, especially the media, but the problem is always the same: you're stuck on your 1st Floor! So, be aware that interacting only on the 1st Floor—exclusively as a family—will disconnect you from your partner, making the "familiarity aspect" very accentuated. To have a truly meaningful relationship, you must "climb the stairs…"

The 2nd Floor, going up! Now you are getting to the 2nd Floor—the hardest level of interaction—where your truths are exposed. Emotional intimacy is the goal for the establishment of a solid 2nd Floor—being emotionally connected. At this point, I want to emphasize the importance of maintaining interactions and communication, between you and your partner, at the same generational level; this means, you and your partner need to communicate as "equals," avoiding the crossing of hierarchical levels by assuming parental roles. Do not pretend to be your partner's parent or offspring! Be just a partner, so that you can be a real romantic couple interacting in all your "floors" in a consistent way, at the same hierarchical level. Otherwise, lovemaking will be extremely difficult, if not impossible, because true passionate love is not possible within dysfunctional hierarchical organizations.

Hierarchies have been defined as the degree of intergenerational boundaries between parents and offspring, or in this case between partners, reflecting the power structure of the family. So, holding your couple relationship as a unit within your family, keeping your boundaries, and differentiating your roles as partners and parents—if you have children—will lead you to healthy interactions, and the possibility, the freedom, and the assurance of enjoying all your "floors"—a family life, a couple life, and a sex life.

Once you can go up and leave your 1st Floor, you can create your 2nd Floor, so you can work on your 3rd Floor easily and have fun. Remember that your 2nd Floor is "the heart" of your relationship—you need to work this out before moving to the 3rd Floor. Once your 2nd Floor is well established, it will be easy to have conversations regularly. Don't panic! Just be together and connected. It is the time dedicated to one another and your love life.

Create now your "couple time"—quality time with your partner (keep yourself from the compulsive Internet, and limit the use of cell phones: calls, video games, texting). Begin dating again. The more skills you have for communication, the better. Problem-solving communication—mostly used on your 1st Floor—is different from emotional communication. In my opinion, the stronger your 2nd Floor is, the stronger your 3rd Floor will be—it's not an absolute but it usually happens. Your "2nd Floor leads to the emotional intimacy you need to be "one" with your partner, to free yourself and *make love 365 times* a year, on your 3rd Floor…

The Three-Floor House model is the best way I have found to explain and create a healthy, functional, satisfactory, stable, passionate, and happy relationship: through positive interactions and expressions at all different levels—family, relational, and sexual—in a consequent and balanced way. Someone who is in a healthy relationship, navigating freely on all three floors, is not afraid. This is something I learned the hard way.

I married my first husband at twenty, and we totally abandoned our 2nd Floor—our couple life—we completely lost it, and of course, we never developed a solid 3rd Floor, even having had three wonderful children. We had no real knowledge or understanding of how the other felt or viewed the world. So, when we faced a major crisis—our "house burned down"—our relationship collapsed, so we could not communicate and discuss what we needed to do any longer. When the chips were down, we each saw who the other really was, and realized we did not know each other at all. When I was finally divorced at age 33, for the first time, I was forced to be on my own and learn about myself. I had to become my best friend and my lover. After a time, I pushed myself to find my real self. And I did!

Then, at age 45, I felt ready to share who I was and to start building a solid 3-Floor House with a lifetime partner somewhere. My second husband, Pedro, was 48, and I was 45 when we married, and we were both eager and ready to fulfill our dreams. And we did! After many years together, we are still in love, in lust, and *making love 365 times a year*! It was not easy at all; we needed to consistently work on building our 2nd Floor—that was the hardest task for us. Nowadays, I believe we have a very solid—Three-Floor House—relationship: strong, reliable, stable, committed, long-lasting, passionate, loving, fulfilling, fun, satisfactory, and healthy for both of us—full of LOVEX!

I know it is possible to have a passionate relationship throughout time, where you can love freely and be loved in the same way and make love as much as you wish. That is why I am sharing this information with you, because I am sure you can do it too!

"Let there be spaces in your togetherness and let
the winds of heavens dance between you."
—Kahlil Gibran

Part V: 7 Simple Suggestions & Recommended Sources

7 Simple Suggestions for Better Expression

1. Consciously build together a solid "Three-Floor House," where level 1 is about having healthy family interactions, Level 2 is about creating emotional intimacy between you and your partner, and Level 3 is about enjoying sexual intimacy in which lovemaking can evolve. Make sure to use different expressions, language, and behaviors in each of the three levels of interaction—your "three floors"—by differentiating each level in your mind, and thus consciously ensuring that you and your partner "feed" each space daily. Remember that it is very easy to get stuck in the 1st Floor, increasing familiarity, forgetting the other spaces by decreasing emotional and sexual intimacy. Having a solid 3rd Floor will ensure you can *make love 365 times a year*!

2. Before you talk or approach your partner, take time to reflect, elaborate, and choose the appropriate words, actions, and facial expressions to turn your partner towards you instead of pushing them away by criticism—because the idea is to find love, not war, in your relationship. Communication between the two of you should be more than words; it involves the establishment of an emotional connection for sexual delight. Always keep this in mind!

3. Do Pretzel Time every morning for at least 10 minutes, as soon as you wake up. Lay together, already naked, and snuggle like a "big pretzel," legs and arms intertwined. Touch each other as much as you can, and kiss, because it will help you produce tons of oxytocin and vasopressin to enhance your connection and trusty bonds.

4. Keep your conversations as assertive and proactive as possible, avoiding loud, aggressive, and impulsive language and expressions, as well as defensiveness and stonewalling. Train yourself in assertiveness by buying books and materials to improve your communication skills. Assertiveness is wisdom! Be aware of what your communicational goal is so that you can successfully communicate to your partner.

5. Discuss your feelings, desires, needs, and ideas in a safe space—therefore building a 2nd Floor is important so you have a space to talk! Don't let negative emotions turn into resentment by keeping them inside of you. Keeping resentment will worsen any situation and may ruin your sex life—your 3rd Floor. Express your feelings using "I," to be able to speak safely and find release, peace, and comfort.

6. Seek professional help if the process of building intimacy becomes too difficult, because professional counseling will provide guidance and continuity as you proactively reach your goal.

7. Take a mirror when you are feeling negative and look at your facial expressions! Be aware of how ugly, hard, and threatening you may look. Choose nice facial expressions to project happiness, even during difficult times or disappointing situations, especially if you are in your 3rd Floor! Inhale, exhale, and relax; the best approach to problem solving is by being calm. Learn to soothe your partner and practice self-soothing. It is the most powerful way to not escalate and to keep your connection in order to *make love 365 times a year*!

Recommended Sources for Sex Secret #4

Assertiveness: How to Stand Up for Yourself and Still Win the Respect of Others by Judy Murphy

The Assertiveness Workbook by Dr. Dena Michelli, Ph.D.

Patryk & Kasia Wezowski: www.centerforbodylanguage.com

Truth & Lies What People are Really Thinking by Dr. Mark Bowden & Tracey Thomson

Dangerous Personalities by Joe Navarro

The Heart of Desire by Stella Resnick, Ph.D.

The Pleasure Zone by Stella Resnick, Ph.D.

Passionate Marriage by David Schnarch, Ph.D.

When fantasy meets reality: Sexual Communication in Relationships by Mike Anderson, TED Talks, June 3, 2015

Profiles Using Indicators of Marital Communication, Communication Styles, and Marital Satisfaction in Mexican Couples by Claudia Bravo, and Alejandra Watty. Journal of Sex and Marital Therapy 43(4): March 2016

Biochemistry of Love by S. Carter, & Porges, S. Noba textbook series: Psychology. Champaign, IL: DEF publishers. 2017

The Loneliness Cure: Six Strategies for Finding Real Connections in Your Life by Floyd, Kory Avon

Hold Me Tight: Seven Conversations for a Lifetime of Love by Sue Johnson

The Science of Touching and Feeling by David Linden, TED Talks, April 8, 2016

SEX SECRET 5

CHAPTER 5

Finding Pleasures

➤+————o+▷

Take your pleasures seriously.

—Charles Eames

"Only when you are in a state of pleasantness,
your body, your mind works at its best."

—Sadhguru

Part I: The Capacity for Pleasure

One of the best quotes I have found that describes pleasure is from Cherie Carter-Scott: "Pleasure is the physical manifestation of joy." Many people, generations, and societies have taken for granted the value of pleasure, minimizing its importance for our overall well-being. In the same way, it has also been exacerbated, leading many to foolishness.

Most of my clients when they first come to my office, as well as people I know, aren't truly thinking about pleasure. Or if they are, they aren't exactly sure what pleasure is, and experience guilt when they have fun and feel joy. While there are many definitions of pleasure, all equate pleasure with a feeling of happy satisfaction and enjoyment. You may derive pleasure from a person, entertainment outside of your work and home life, your inner self, or an activity like sex. But the key to this definition is one word: happiness!

Happiness is connected to pleasure, and pleasure is connected to sexuality. You should first understand how to be happy before you can experience real pleasure. Scientists used to think of happiness as an abstract idea, something fanciful, ephemeral, with no factual evidence, therefore; not something that could be worked on. Nowadays, new research has shown that we can work on happiness! Happiness is a fact. It is a skill that can be improved like any other.

If you don't have a pleasurable life, how will you have a pleasurable sex life? Recall the Three-Floor House from the last chapter. You must build a good foundation before you can fully work on your sex life. So, look for little pleasures outside of the bedroom first; enjoy being in the here and now. You don't want to be in a movie theatre and so are worried about what you're doing after, or if you get a good parking spot you are worried that you will miss the movie. Life is the same way! You need to be focused on the present moment to enjoy it. What are the pleasures you can add to your life to build your 1st Floor as a family? Take time to have a glass of wine with friends, play with your kids, learn a new skill. This pleasure has some limits—social constraints you must be aware of. Then you can work on your 2nd Floor—time with your partner. Take time for dates, talking, walks, or playing games together. Here you will have more freedom and less control within the safety of your partner. You need both of these "Floors."

My point is that if you don't have pleasure in Level 1 and 2, how, according to the model, will you have pleasure in Level 3? So please, open your mind to pleasure. You cannot have a healthy sex life without pleasure. Remember that healthy sex is sex you have for pleasure. This is one of the criteria for sex to be considered healthy sex. If you are having sex out of duty, obligation, or manipulation, it isn't healthy. Lovemaking is all about pleasure and connection! Please refer to Chapter 3.

But to do this, you must understand happiness and pleasure first. Build up your capacity for experiencing happiness and pleasure in your normal life to access the freedom of expressing your needs for sexual pleasure. Author Jon Leiss points out that "the capacity to have pleasure is part of being healthy." Let's see below two cases that illustrate the importance of pleasure in life. Then, you will see Mahid and Joya's Lovemaking Wheels.

Cases # 5: Mahid & Joya and Henry & Vivian

Once again, we are going to look at two cases with two very different couples but very similar problems. This is to show how lack of pleasure affects relationships, something that can happen to anyone wrapped blindly in everyday life! While both couples have good relationships and love each other, they are from different cultures, different religions, and are different ages. But in both cases, the women struggle with a lack of pleasure in their sex life.

First, let's look at Mahid and Joya. Joya is 30 years old, and Mahid is 31. They have a 7-year-old son. Both are successful in their careers and love one another without carrying any resentment.

Second are Henry and Vivian. She is 45 years old, and he is 47. They have three boys between the ages of 5 and 12. Like Mahid and Joya, they are successful and have no resentment. In both cases the women were raised in an overprotected environment and are constantly worried about caring for their mothers. During their childhood their mothers took too much care of them, and now they are expected to reciprocate this.

When I first met Joya, she came to see me alone. Her first statement told me what I needed to know: "I have a lot of anxiety; it is very hard for me to relax and enjoy. I don't know how to be happy."

I asked her to elaborate.

"I have too much anxiety. Then I feel nervous and am only thinking about the pain and problems in my life; then my anxiety gets worse. Then I think of more problems and just go numb."

She told me she knew Mahid loved her and he had her see her family doctor.

"All the tests are okay, but I feel overtired and don't want to do anything besides my work and duties at home. I am very responsible."

Throughout the session, she had a very serious, blank, apathetic expression on her face. I asked about hobbies, and she told me: "I don't have any hobbies, nor pleasurable activities. I don't allow myself."

Joya's mother was overbearing and constantly worried about keeping her daughter from danger. She saw worries and concerns around every corner. Heights, fun, sex: these were all causes for high anxiety. In her eyes, "pleasure was bad, having fun was irresponsible, and happiness a fairytale." Now Joya couldn't enjoy anything, including sex with Mahid.

"Nothing entertains me, nothing pleases me," she explained to me.

I asked about her frequency of masturbation since her sex rate was so low, but she didn't do this either. "It's impossible," she told me. She had "no pleasure in life and no pleasure in sex, and no time for that thing…" Even though she believed sexuality was healthy and important, she was unable to "act" on her desires.

Vivian, however, was obsessed with not wasting time. She was raised to see any kind of pleasure as a timewaster; she only did things for her husband and kids. In her perfectionistic eyes, everything she did was a duty that had to be done "right." When she and Henry came to see me, Vivian started the conversation.

"I don't know what happened to me."

Henry jumped in, saying, "my purpose in being here is to move forward because we seem stuck. I want to improve our relationship, but nothing pleases her. She's very apathetic, especially in bed."

As with all my clients, I made sure to talk to Vivian alone to establish that there was no hidden resentment or latent health issues. She was physically active, and she and Henry communicated well. But she could not find any pleasure in life. She only went out for him; the whole time, she simply wished to be home so that she could focus on her tasks.

"We can't even go see a movie," Henry complained. "She sees it as a waste of time and refuses to go."

"I'm not used to enjoyment," Vivian said. "I'm too worried about the kids, the house, and work." Vivian could not stop herself from working, in and out of the home.

"I know my husband is frustrated," she continued. She still had a very low desire for sex, even though she believed it was important, but couldn't act on it—the same as Joya.

In both cases, the women made themselves very tired by completing tasks so that they could avoid a fun time. They avoided sex as well, because sexual activities are about pleasure and relaxation. Even further, they avoided having pleasure of any kind.

Everything seemed to be a chore for them, even lovemaking—for different reasons. Now both had sad and angry husbands. Any sex they had was bad sex because the women were enjoying it all. Joya was only focused on her fears; Vivian was focused on what tasks she had to do next. Neither received any pleasure out of life nor any pleasure out of sex.

In both instances, the kids were getting older. I frequently notice this when problems suddenly arise in relationships. The problems have been there for longer, but because life is now starting to settle down as children become more independent, these couples begin to once again have more time together, without distractions, so they start realizing how apart and disconnected they are. They also notice the inability they have for experiencing pleasure in their love life. Now they know what they have been missing…

The following are Mahid and Joya's Lovemaking Wheels. See how low they both scored in the area of pleasure, Sex Secret #5:

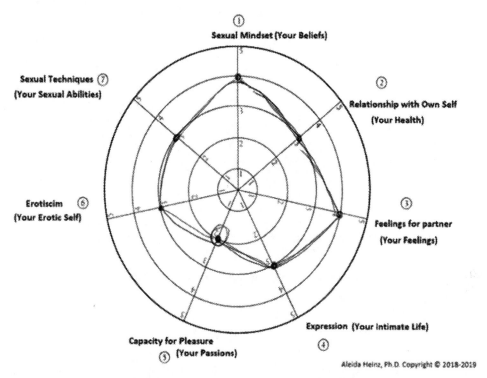

Mahid's Lovemaking Wheel. Wheel #9

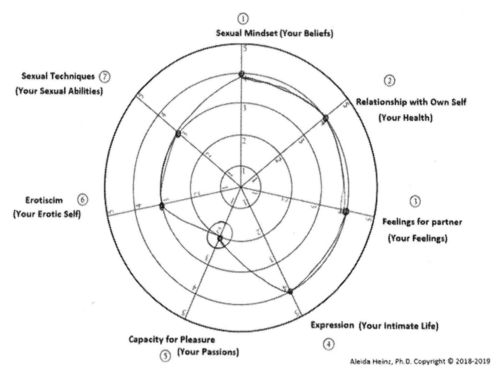

Joya's Lovemaking Wheel. Wheel #10

Another Duo: Happiness & Pleasure

Studies have been done on happiness, demonstrating that it actually exists and can be worked on. So, being happy largely depends on oneself. It is no longer an ephemeral ideal, nor a dream, a fantasy, or a fairytale; it is a fact! Groundbreaking research on happiness was done by psychologist and University of California professor of psychology Sonja Lyubomirsky, PhD, who has pioneered the scientific understanding of happiness and has provided us a detailed way to increase it, based on a large quantity of experimental data.

Lyubomirsky has researched the possibility of permanently increasing happiness. She was honored with the Diener Award for Outstanding Midcareer, the UC Riverside Distinguished Research Lecturer Award, a Templeton Positive Psychology Prize, a Science of Generosity grant, two John Templeton Foundation grants, a Character Lab grant, a Psychology & Philosophy grant, and a million-dollar grant from the National Institute of Mental Health. Outstanding! So, there is no doubt about her findings on happiness, proving that happiness is a fact, so that we all can make ourselves happier if we want.

According to Lyubomirsky's findings—known as the "50-10-40% Formula," or—in Lyubomirsky's words, "the 40% Solution" —our happiness is split into three parts. The first part, "50," makes up 50% of our happiness. This 50% is in our genetics. You cannot change this. The genetic predisposition to be happy may be seen in babies; for instance, I have three children, and I believe that my oldest son is naturally happy because he was born laughing! It is amazing to see how easily he laughed at people, and still does—I'm sure he has an internal disposition to smile and feel happy. To my knowledge, no one can measure your "happiness" genes, but whatever level you are naturally happy at, that is your level.

Since you cannot change this first half, it makes sense to work on what you can change—the second half. The second half is workable, and it is broken into two parts: the 10% and the 40%. The 10% is everything around you, the outside and external circumstances in your life such as your family, relationships, work, and money, etc., which are partly—not totally—under your control; that is, only 50% of this 10% can be under your control. It is about the good and bad things that happen to us in life. Have you won the lottery? Have you enjoyed great times with your partner? Happiness! Does your roof leak and must be replaced? Have you been fired? Did your partner leave you? Unhappiness…

Unfortunately, this is what most people focus on when working to be happy, trying to control 100% in vain. You cannot control the events that happen in your life, especially the negative ones. You cannot even control others in your life. You can only work on improving your relationships and getting successful by changing or improving your own self, no one else, so it is always a partial work. What you can only do is to control your reactions to events, not the events per se! In other words, your mind is the only piece you can work on and control 100%—that's it! Not your life circumstances.

The last and most important part of your happiness, the 40%—your "40% Solution" —depends only on your mindset. It is about your thoughts and behavior. In turn, this part is sub divided in half, 20% is about your conscious thoughts, and 20% is about your actions, the things you do in life. The activities you choose can bring you different pleasures. If you love playing tennis, make time in your life to play tennis. This makes a difference in your happiness level. Lyubomirsky says, "this much happiness—up to 40%—is within your power to change; if you are prepared to do the work."

Remember from Chapter 1, how your mindset is key to everything. You need to ditch your ANTs (Automatic Negative Thoughts). No one else can change your mindset; this is entirely up to you, which is why creating a positive sexual mindset is the first step in this book! Your mindset is not influenced by events; it changes your interpretation of events. By being aware of your own thoughts that led to your actions, and choosing them right and to your favor, you will become much happier! Some people believe having a partner will make them happy, or that their partner should make them happy. This is the same as staking your happiness on winning the lottery. Do not let your happiness depend on outside factors! Unless you are incredibly lucky, this won't make you happy. Instead of focusing on the 10%, work on the 40% you can control.

Pleasure

Recall that mind and brain are intertwined. So, what role does the brain play in pleasure? A huge role! Pleasure comes from a complex set of circuitries in your brain, particularly in the orbital frontal cortex. Scientists have observed that the neurological pathways in the front part of the brain, become very active when we engage in pleasurable activities, such as eating sweet and fatty foods, shopping, and of course, experiencing orgasms!

The pleasure circuit is crucial to enjoying fun activities, feeling pleasure, and feeling rewarded. By allowing ourselves to experience pleasure and feel rewarded, our motivation is strengthened, our mood improves, and we experience happiness. Robert Maleenka, who I have spoken about before, says, "if this circuitry is working properly, it doles out pleasure when achieving a desirable goal or experience, like food or sex. If it doesn't, anhedonia is the result." This circuitry breaking down will keep you from pleasure, even keep you from seeking pleasure, making you feel unhappy instead. We will discuss this phenomenon more in the next section.

As you pursue pleasure, you will come up with two principles. The first is the Pleasure Principle, which is an automatic mental drive or instinct seeking to avoid pain and obtain pleasure and happiness. Its counterpart, the Reality Principle, is a learning process to regulate and temper our pleasures. Both are important to sustaining a healthy life. The Pleasure Principle is related to wanting and liking— "I want!" "I want you!" The easiest place to see this is in a child. They have not yet learned the Reality Principle and are all about desire: "I like it," "I want more," "I want this." There is no regulation. If you let a two-year-old eat candy, they usually won't stop until they are sick. They have not yet learned how to temper their desires.

With the Reality Principle, the natural reaction is "I don't like," "I don't need," "I should not," "I must," "I must not." It is all about avoiding pleasure and fun. The reality principle keeps us from going to extremes; the pursuit of too much pleasure can lead to addiction. The reality principle usually brings balance, but those stuck with only the reality principle may find no pleasure, fun, or happiness at all. Those living only on the reality principle often suffer from low sexual desire, for instance. And it makes sense! The desire for sex is a desire for pleasure.

It is good to have some control, but not too much, so you're able to enjoy yourself and have fun. You must be able to let go and to control your pleasures. Seek activities that will help you meet the demands of the external world—those you will encounter in your family, community, work, etc. Remember that regularly doing activities you enjoy can increase your happiness by 20%! Using the Reality Principle to choose the best activities for you will help you consciously seek activities that please you. This will give you the happiness and serenity to deal with the rest of your responsibilities.

As American writer and lecturer Dale Carnegie said, "people rarely succeed unless they have fun in what they are doing. Happiness doesn't depend on any external conditions; it is governed by our mental attitude. One of the most tragic things I know about human nature is that all of us tend to put off living." Often society will impose rules on pleasure for controlling its people. This leads to a "socially created reality principle." Sometimes this can be good, but other times, societal pressures can lead to a repression of pleasure to meet the external expectations of governmental and religious organizations. So, make sure you are consciously doing what works best for your overall well-being. Everything in life needs a balance! Balance is healthy.

Imbalance leads to depression and anxiety—either by excess or scarcity. I have noticed that in America, there is an abundance of depression and anxiety, maybe due to society's suppression of pleasures. We've talked before about demands society places on people to focus more on work and success than on pleasure, love, and relationships. This is the Reality Principle in overdrive! If you belong to a religious organization, be aware of the role your religion is playing in the suppression of your pleasure, especially sexual pleasure. As author Daniel Willey says, "I am fascinated at how much time we spend doing things that we don't enjoy." Be aware of your thoughts and your actions, are they bringing you joy, pleasure, and happiness? Just be wise! As long as you find true joy in your activities and practices, it's great!

How could you *make love 365 times a year* without first knowing how to enjoy the little things in your life, and without knowing how to take time to relax and have fun?

It is transcendent to understand the importance of happiness and pleasure to our well-being. According to Beecham, from previous chapters, optimal performance is being "in the zone or the flow." It is, to me, as being in a "zone of happiness and pleasure." Beecham states that "dopamine, endorphins, and anandamide are the three neurochemicals that are most associated with flow, and they are critical to happiness and optimal functioning." Balancing the Reality Principle and the Pleasure Principle is, in my opinion, the greatest challenge we face in Western society. This is especially true for sexual pleasure. So, how to make sure you are balancing correctly—not too much, not too little?

Part II: Too Little: Lack of Pleasure—Anhedonia

The more capacity you have in order to feel pleasure and enjoy it, the more capacity you will have to enjoy your sex life. We have seen the importance of pleasure for our well-being. But what happens when you don't have pleasure on any level of your life? Lack of pleasure is a real mental health problem known as anhedonia. The word anhedonia literally comes from the Greek "an," which means "without," and "hedone," which means pleasure. Those who suffer from anhedonia—the inability to experience pleasure—find it hard to relax and have fun in their daily lives. They either cannot or will not seek pleasurable activities and will stick instead to duties and stress.

I agree with psychotherapist Anita Gadhia-Smith in that some people simply do not believe pleasure is important or are unable to experience it for diverse reasons such as intense repressed feelings like loss, betrayal, and anger. Also, it can be a symptom, as Michael D. McGee, Chief Medical Officer of The Haven at Pismo California says, of many disorders: "clinical depression, bipolar disorder, childhood trauma, substance misuse, post-traumatic stress disorder and difficult but temporary life circumstances, such as a divorce, the death of a loved one or job loss."

However, medical researchers don't know what causes anhedonia, according to Gabriel S. Dichter, an associate Professor of Psychiatry and Psychology at the University of North Carolina School of Medicine. Ask for professional help if you think you are not experiencing pleasure often, at least in the things you used to enjoy. Anhedonia, according to Stanford University Medical Center, is a "major source of depression," associated with no feelings of joy, a dull life, unhappiness, anxiety, low sexual desire, and chronic stress. It's the loss of the ability to have fun, the loss of even tactile pleasures such as touch and taste. Sufferers have a diminished interest in engaging in activities other than duties, work, and chores.

In Western Judeo-Christian culture, suffering is valued and seen as important to be a "good person." This does not do pleasure any favors. Think about it! Usually, I observe that a suffering person is more accepted and validated than a person who enjoys the pleasures of life. People I interview often say it is okay for them to cry a lot in privacy, but not okay to masturbate—that is, experience pleasure. In our culture, suffering is better than pleasure. And as people begin to think that not having pleasure is okay, they start to see having no pleasure as the norm. Moreover, as I said before, commonly in America the aim is work and money. It is a materialistic and individualistic society—as reviewed in previous chapters—it is not a society that values pleasure. This may lead to the self-denial of personal pleasures, even sometimes distrusting them by feeling guilty when experiencing leisure time, as in the cases of Joya and Vivian.

"When our ability to enjoy pleasure in a particular area is limited, excitement can be interpreted negatively and bring up fearful thoughts and feelings. Excitement turns into fear and feels terribly uncomfortable," explains Resnick. People deny pleasures rather than enjoy them, because, unfortunately, we have been trained to resist pleasure in our lives, as explained in *The Pleasure Zone*. In fact, pleasure is not only important but essential! Pleasure supports our mental health and bolsters our immune system, according to recent studies. There is no evidence that pleasure contributes to illness, mental weaknesses, or social or moral declines. By saying that pleasure is an enemy, society is reaching back to Puritan doctrine that considered a soul experiencing pleasure to be an "at risk" soul. Thanks to it, pleasure is heavily associated with guilt. To find happiness, you must learn to balance your pleasurable activities without guilt.

This is the problem Joya faced. Her mother had ingrained in her that feeling pleasure was wrong, so fun activities just brought guilt on her. She needed to first reset her mindset about pleasure before she could move forward! Her negative view of pleasure, fun, relaxation, and leisure time kept her from feeling anything besides guilt. And of course, with guilt comes depression and anxiety. Anhedonia and related depression decrease our overall quality of life. And, 1 in 5 Americans suffer from depression! Anhedonia causes depression, and depression causes chronic stress. This chronic stress leads to more depression, the depression leads to anhedonia, and anhedonia leads to more stress. It's a bad cycle! And our society is very much caught up in causing chronic stress. It has been shown that chronic stress leads to the inability to have pleasure—which includes sexual pleasure. Lack of sexual pleasure will cause you to stop having sex, and now the cycle is even bigger and stronger.

What a trap!

In my opinion, Vivian could have been suffering from anhedonia. The chronic stresses in her life had weighed her down to the degree that she no longer knew how to look for pleasure. Happiness had become a foreign concept, and her constant stress now felt normal. But, fortunately, not to her husband! Thanks to his complaint, they started doing something about it and improving their relationship and sex life. Now, they are aware of this fatal trap!

You must wisely manage stress and pointless suffering to find happiness and pleasure in your life, and of course, in your love life! Healthy sex is one of those pleasurable activities that can bring you happiness. But it will be very difficult to have a healthy sex life and *make love 365 times a year* if you suffer from anhedonia—having sex as a duty with no pleasure isn't healthy. Dr. David A. Kalmbach of Kent University found that "anhedonia depression was more uniquely related to most sexual problems among women." Most women's sexual problems relate to touch, so no wonder this lack of pleasure is the cause! Dr. Julia Warnock, University of Oklahoma, took the study farther when she found that a third of adult women in the U.S. suffer from low sexual desire and disinterest in pleasure. The central feature in her study saw a deficit of sexual fantasies and desire for sexual encounters, fantasies, and desire that could help counter their chronic stress.

Anhedonia in our lives can lead to sexual anhedonia. In males, this is also known as "ejaculatory anhedonia," where men ejaculate with no pleasure. It's a physical sensation with no mental feelings whatsoever. In women, sexual anhedonia is a lack of pleasure, even during orgasm. If you suffer from anhedonia because of stress, a busy life, or depression, then you may not be motivated to have sex at all. And, if you do engage in sexual activities, it is probably for the wrong reasons. A way to bring pleasure back into your life is by starting small. Bring small pleasures back into your everyday life: relax, be still, enjoy being alive, and recognize what brings you happiness. Doing yoga or working out may help you regain pleasure again. Experience these small steps without guilt. It is important to experience pleasure in life so you can experience pleasure in sex.

Find professional help as soon as possible. Even those not experiencing anhedonia can benefit from bringing more pleasure into their life; open yourself to experiencing joy, fun, happiness, and pleasure! Talk to your partner about it. Find pleasure with your partner. As author Terri Guillemets says, "pleasure and discipline need to stay close friends."

Part III: Too Much: The Dark Side of Pleasure—Addiction

On the other hand, is it possible to have too much pleasure? According to science, yes, and it, in turn, will eventually become unpleasant. As an ancient hedonistic philosopher, Aristippus of Cyrene, said, "the best thing is to possess pleasures without being their slave, not to be devoid of pleasures." Addiction usually stems from trying to avoid emotional pain through extreme measures—usually with excess of alcohol, drugs, sex, or food. It is the Pleasure Principle in overdrive! As we've discussed, pleasure is a pendulum. In one direction you find anhedonia, no pleasure, and in the opposite direction, you find the danger of swinging too far the other way—reaching the point of addiction: the dark side of pleasure, according to John Hopkins University neuroscientist Dr. David J. Linden.

Imagine pleasure as a spectrum: you have one side with no color at all, the overcontrolled-restricted-zone—anhedonia—while the opposite side is all black and dark, the uncontrolled-out of control-zone—addiction. The idea is to be in a bright "orange zone," at the absolute middle of the spectrum: healthy pleasure balanced with an exquisite equilibrium between fun, happiness, and diligence, between "colors," without being a slave...

Dr. Linden points out that memory and pleasure are closely intertwined, so "pleasure is central to learning." He states that "most experiences in our lives that we find transcendent—whether illicit vices or socially sanctioned rituals and social practices as diverse as exercise or even charitable giving—activate an anatomically and biochemically defined pleasure circuit in the brain." That means, many of the activities we do, positive or negative, can activate the pleasure circuit, making us feel good; others don't, and we have learned that. Linden explains that "this intrinsic pleasure circuitry can also be co-opted by artificial activators like cocaine or nicotine or heroin or alcohol…these particular neurons also compromise another battleground. The dark side of pleasure, of course, is an addiction."

Furthermore, Linden also explains that "they actually seem to want it more but like it less." This source of activities and substances that activate the circuit pleasure in the brain can lead us to feel great but also can become compulsive. One example is drug addictions. Here did the pleasure go if you don't like it anymore? If something becomes unpleasant, it is not good either, right?

The World Health Organization (WHO) describes addiction as "repeated use of a psychoactive substance or substances, to the extent that the user (referred to as an addict) is periodically or chronically intoxicated, shows a compulsion to take the preferred substance (or substances), has great difficulty in voluntarily ceasing or modifying substance use, and exhibits determination to obtain psychoactive substances by almost any means." As their study of addiction has continued, they have introduced the word "dependence" into the definition as well and have broadened their idea of substance dependence to include "psychosocial, environmental, biological and genetic factors," finding that the brain plays a large role in dependence.

There are many different views about whether addiction can refer to an activity, rather than a substance. Or even if there is such a thing as too much sex! These different viewpoints can be broken down into:

1. Moral vs. immoral model: This model assumes that a life devoted to pleasure is lacking in value and sees anyone who seeks sex for pure pleasure as immoral; that person's goals and values are bad and weak. It sees addiction as morally weak.
2. The Brain-disease model: These are people who see addictions as brain damage. Addiction is seen as an involuntary, mental, and neurological problem. The brain-disease model, according to Drs. Satel & Lilienfeld, "obscures the dimension of choice in addiction, the capacity to respond to incentives, and also the essential fact people use drugs for reasons."
3. The Liberal view: This view is more optimistic and sees distinctions in pleasures. This is the view that correlates pleasure and addiction. Addiction is seen as a choice that inevitably changes brain functioning.

The first and second viewpoints are negative ideas of addiction, and this is how addiction was viewed for most of history. Studies have been done to verify if pleasure is the objective of addiction. One of these studies concluded that we should err the side of caution by taking at face value the behavior of drug addicts—they are rational choosers who value drugs for their rewarding properties more than they value the alternatives. Therefore, studies on addiction have concluded that it is a matter of acting on one's strong appetitive desires for pleasure, and that is all.

The World Health Organization says addiction is the "repeated use of substances along with a compulsion to take them." The Diagnostic and Statistical Manual of Mental Disorders (DSM–5), used to categorize mental disorders, claims there are behavioral addictions as well, a compulsion to engage in certain acts that will lead to psychological pleasure. Harmful consequences can also come from these behavioral addictions—when they become compulsive. We may conclude that having pleasure is healthy and good as long as it doesn't become compulsive. But what is the meaning of compulsion? How can we become compulsive? What is the line? What is your line?

Compulsion comes from the Latin "compellere," "to drive," "a force." Compulsion is the action or state of forcing or being forced to do something and an irresistible urge to behave in a certain way, especially against one's conscious wishes." As Linden says, "you want it more but like it less." The pleasure is gone, but the need is still there, and growing fast, because probably you have learned only one way—an unhealthy way—to activate the pleasure circuitry in your brain.

Sex Addiction

Does sex addiction exist? Is there such a thing as too much sex? What about *making love 365 times a year*—is it an addiction? A compulsion? It is NOT! Let's review it well so that you can be sure, safe, secure, comfortable, and confident about *making love 365 times a year* without, thinking you are a freak! Lovemaking is NOT, and cannot be, an addiction or a compulsion, even if you make love every day. Let's explore what would be an addiction.

Know first that the topic this very controversial. The controversy is over if substance and behavioral addictions exist, and if they are equals. A case can be made for both sides, as this is a heavy topic that is not always clear, especially for sex: sex compulsion or sex addiction? Most psychologists, though, believe that behavioral addictions are real and need to be addressed. Sex is a behavior; however, as the American Association of Sexuality Educators, Counselors and Therapists (AASECT) stipules, there is not "sufficient empirical evidence to support the classification of sex addition or porn addiction as a mental health disorder."

Therefore, sex addiction is still a complicated subject. Many recognize and know—as I do—healthy sex as a positive behavior which does not bring any negative consequences or problems. Keep in mind that I am referring to the HEALTHY sex—you can review healthy sex in Chapter 2. Any uncontrolled sexual behavior—addition or compulsion—is not healthy, and it must be labeled as unhealthy sex, not just "sex." Addiction formation may happen when you overdo something very pleasurable, with no control, especially for highly addictive substances. This can happen with almost any activity—eating, sex, shopping, gambling, working, the Internet, etc. Moreover, it seems that certain activities, food, and substances also have different degrees of addictive properties; some are higher, while others are less addictive, making you want more to light up that pleasure sensation.

The thing is that you will want more and more of "that," but the dopamine that was produced will decrease, and you will no longer feel so good, but the "need" will persist. Therefore, you will end up hating what you did, but still need it without being able to stop! This is what happens with addictions. You depend on the substance or behavior without wishing for it, eliminating the possibilities for real pleasure. Along this line of thinking, Linden continues, "in a way a symptom of the concept of sex addiction is similar to the problems of food and addiction and obesity." Now we have to ask, when does behavior become an addiction?

The criteria are no different than for drugs or alcohol:

▶ Negative life consequences.
▶ The behavior becomes necessary to feel "normal."
▶ Broken promises.
▶ Feelings of remorse—no more pleasure, just "unwanted necessity."

Remember the definitions of compulsion? The state of forcing and not thinking; an urge to behave against one's conscious wishes, so it is something you really do not want to do any more but cannot control; it is compulsive: there is no thinking but acting on needs. There is nothing healthy about this! The pleasure is gone, and your willpower as well. Therefore, sexual activities done under these circumstances—uncontrolled, compulsive— are unhealthy.

Lovemaking vs. Unhealthy Sex

Lovemaking, on the other hand, is ALWAYS healthy because it does not come from compulsion, or an uncontrolled impulse, caused by a mere sexual need, and then, as a result, feelings of guilt, emptiness, and regret, instead of real pleasure. Remember that true lovemaking is always about love, connection, and pleasure—both parties agree, want to, like, and enjoy engaging in this "sharing" activity in a safe, joyful and risk-free space. Lovemaking has no room for manipulation, urges, personal interest, objectifications, or compulsions. There is nothing that can be compared to the act of lovemaking and being connected at all levels.

Therefore, unhealthy, compulsive sex has nothing to do with lovemaking. Linden is one of the leading psychologists who sees sex addiction as a real problem, painful and unpleasant. In *The Compass of Pleasure*, Linden says that "sex addicts" have the same problems as other addicts; more and more sex is necessary for them to achieve pleasure, and they may destroy themselves to feel this sensation over and over. This is not healthy, and this is NOT about lovemaking; it is about compulsive and risky sex, where, according to Linden, "you need more but like it less…"

The American Association of Sexuality Educators, Counselors, and Therapists "does not find the sexual addiction training and treatment methods and educational pedagogies to be adequately informed by accurate human sexuality knowledge." Therefore, these unclear ideas of sexual addiction can lead to further repression and more misunderstandings regarding healthy sexuality. Furthermore, any addiction, whether substance or behavioral, should be addressed by an expert professional so you can grow into your best self! If sex is becoming "a problem" for you, either in lacking or excess, underlying problems need to be addressed—do not just label the problem, avoid it, or blame yourself or others. If you are engaging in any action that harms you or your loved ones, you need to find help immediately!

My view about "sex addiction" is that it isn't a sexual problem—it is a control problem!

Now, how to keep ourselves happy and experiencing pleasure regularly?

How to be sure we are not crossing the line between healthy pleasure and unhealthiness? How do we know when it is too little or too much?

Sexual Pleasure

Health is related to pleasure, and pleasure is related to desire, and desire is related to sexuality, including sexual pleasure. Let's talk about sexual pleasure, a fundamental element to *making love 365 times a year.* Why is that? Because, if you find real pleasure in your sexual experiences, you are more likely to repeat this again and again—not compulsively and uncontrollably, but consciously—to experience joy in every encounter... The opposite is also true; if you are not having pleasure when your partner touches you the way you like to be touched, it may be a sign that something is going on, something either about yourself or your relationship. Always remember that lovemaking is about love, pleasure, freedom, and connection.

By now you should know what pleasure is, and its importance. Now I want you to understand intense pleasures such as sexual pleasure, which has nothing to do with addiction or compulsion, although they might seem close to each other. I believe that a passionless life is when you become engrossed in meaningless duties and routines, feeling bored, sad, no very active with low energy, and even depressed. Just because you have some ordinary pleasures and enjoy your routine, you are not necessarily living with passion and experiencing intense pleasures. In essence, there is nothing wrong with that, but you are missing the fierce joys to live with passion!

So, is sexual pleasure that important? ABSOLUTELY, YES!

In fact, sexual desire depends on sexual pleasure to reinforce it positively, encouraging you to repeat it as I mentioned before. Many couples I see have lots of pleasure in their life, but no sexual pleasure. Why does this happen? It would be hard to have sexual pleasure if you were not experiencing general pleasure in your life, but the reverse happens as well. Individuals who see sexual pleasure as "unnecessary" are missing the opportunity to enjoy their sexuality in a healthy way. This often happens in long-term relationships because these couples no longer have sex for fun and pleasure, so the simple idea of having sex stresses them.

I think we have underestimated how the lack of sexual pleasure can negatively impact our life and our long-term relationships. If the genuine desire for pleasure shapes a woman's pleasure, can she really want a sexless marriage? Would we have such a high divorce rate if pleasure wasn't missing? Think back to your first sexual experience. Was it negative? A study was done with girls in America ages 12-25 and girls in the Netherlands, also 12-25 years old, asking if they enjoyed and had fun during their first sexual experience. Netherland girls, in a school system that advocates knowledge about sexual pleasure, and openness of sexual discussion, had fun and spoke positively about their experiences.

In contrast, 66% or TWO-THIRDS of American girls wished they had waited longer to have sex because their first experiences were negative. The lack of education about sexual pleasure set adults. If you start with negative experiences and fears, you will hold on to that your whole life, if you don't become aware of it. So, how can you then later build a pleasure space with your partner? We must change how we discuss sex in America, especially with teens. We must teach them, and ourselves, how to balance responsibility and pleasure, instead of instilling fear. Then we have changed the dialogue and created another sexual story.

In 2019, the 24th World Association for Sexual Health Congress was held in Mexico City—as I mentioned in Chapter 2. The declaration on Sexual Pleasure was the conclusion of this congress. As I said before, the main theme and emphasis of the congress was the recognition of sexual pleasure as an essential element for our well-being. It was asserted that sexual pleasure is a central part of our existence and our sexual health. Sexual pleasure belongs to our list of human rights, and it is our right to enjoy it freely and healthily. It was emphasized that nobody is obliged to have sexual pleasure; however, it is important that it be considered as an integral part of humanity for a healthier and happier society.

According to the definition given by the World Association for Sexual Health (WAS), "sexual pleasure is the physical and/or psychological satisfaction and enjoyment derived from shared or solitary erotic experiences, including thoughts, fantasies, dreams, emotions, and feelings." You can find the complete declaration of sexual pleasure, as well as more information, in the World Association for Sexual Health website: https://worldsexualhealth.net/declaration-on-sexual-pleasure/

Finding Sexual Pleasure

To experience pleasure in the bedroom is essential to increase desire—to want it more—and to continue doing it. Without feeling pleasant sensations, how will you have the desire to try again? Think about delicious chocolate (I love chocolates!); you taste it and enjoy it, so you experience pleasure eating chocolate—then, next time, you want it more. The more you enjoy it, the more you desire it. You want to experience such a delightful pleasure again. The same happens in bed...

Therefore, enhancing the experience, and feeling comfortable and relaxed, are key to experience sexual pleasure. For instance, in a study done by Herbenick, D., Fu, T., Arter, J., Sanders, S.A. & Dodge, B. in 2017, it was reported that around 40% of women need clitoral stimulation to orgasm, and about the same percent reported that even if they did not need clitoral stimulation to orgasm, it made the experience more pleasurable. Find ways to make your experience more and more pleasurable.

Once again, if you are having problems, review your Lovemaking Wheel to find out what is going on, and work on it—a specific chapter may help you solve the specific problem—because, how can you experience pleasure if it isn't fun? Make it fun and easy! If you are not enjoying your partner, you need to evaluate your feelings carefully. Go back to previous chapters and work on other issues first. What are the reasons for the lack of sexual pleasure? It's always a combination of:

▶ Boredom, lack of sexual knowledge and/or novelty
▶ Limiting physical and/or mental conditions
▶ Spiritual guilt and negative past experiences
▶ Mental block and lack of imagination, curiosity, and creativity
▶ Emotional breakdowns

If you are not having sexual pleasure, then you will be having less and less sex. You are not activating the pleasure circuitry in the brain to bring about dopamine and the pleasure it causes, so you have less incentive to have sex. Women, especially, will begin to have sex out of a sense of duty, to please or reassure their partner. They will still engage in the act but will not enjoy it. Fear of pregnancy and/or STDs can also lead to a lack of sexual fun and may prevent couples from experiencing sexual pleasure. Governments, schools, and religious institutions only impart "negative sex education," so people have become afraid of sex. Young people have learned to fear sex; they need now to learn that sexual pleasure is important, essential, and healthy.

Peggy Orenstein, an expert on women's issues says that "while young women may feel entitled to engage in sexual behavior, they don't necessarily feel entitled to enjoy it." Women's genitals are directly tied to a women's enjoyment of sex, and teens are not taught how their genitals work or how they can be used for pleasure. Therefore, women don't feel that they deserve sexual pleasure, or that only men experience or deserve it. Frequently, the woman's mindset is—especially at an early age—set on pleasing their partners, while most men's is on pleasure for themselves. The key is that everyone becomes responsible for their own pleasure to share it, so that each participant can experience fun, pleasure, and satisfaction.

In fact, young women are more likely than young men to use their partner's pleasure to measure their own satisfaction: "if he is sexually satisfied, then I am," according to University of Michigan professor Sara McClelland. Meanwhile, men are more likely to measure their satisfaction by their own orgasm or how they ejaculate. "Sometimes, women were more focused on pleasing their partners than on maximizing their own erotic fulfillment," says McClelland. So, low desire isn't about missing hormones, but about missing "fun!"

For instance, imagine you don't like going to the beach. You find it dirty, crowded, and too hot. Why would you desire a trip to the coast? You wouldn't! You'd do everything in your power to avoid visiting there. Similarly, if you don't like a certain food, like raw broccoli, you aren't going to shop for it under your own volition. In my opinion, the lack of sexual pleasure is the root of sexual disinterest and low sexual desire.

Jenny Higgins and Jennifer S. Hirsch did a study that found that "sexual health research within public health has largely failed to explore how pleasure and positive sexual functioning affect sexual risk and risk-reduction practices." Their study focused on pleasure and inequality between partners. They made three interesting points, where both women and men reported multiple aspects of enjoyment, of which physical pleasure was only one. Also, a clear link was found between the forms of pleasure respondents seek and their contraceptive practices. They concluded that the more you enjoy sex, the more responsible you will be! The study found that:

1. Pleasure varies
2. Pleasure matters
3. Pleasure intersects with power and social inequality

Furthermore, Higgins and Hirsch found some important factors to be aware of that deeply impact sexual pleasure in women of all ages. They are weight gain, vaginal bleeding, vaginal dryness, body image, and side effects of pills and contraceptive.

- ▶ Weight gain: When a woman does not feel sexy, she stops having fun in bed. Most likely she won't initiate sexual approach! As soon as a woman starts losing some weight and feeling better, she starts feeling sexy again. Period! Get back to Chapter 2.
- ▶ Vaginal bleeding/cramps/physical problems: This normal monthly event is painful for some women; it is not sexy at all, so it is not fun! Just relax and wait! Do it in the shower if you feel like having sex. Follow your instincts…
- ▶ Vaginal dryness: Especially with age, women start worrying about not getting wet enough for intercourse, which is normal. That is why I recommend always having lubricants next to your bed, regardless of your age. There is nothing wrong with the use of lubricants. There is no need worry anymore; just use plenty of lubrication each time you want to go "playing" with your partner.
- ▶ Poor body image: Usually, but not necessarily, this is related to weight gain. Body image is beyond weight; it is about self-love. Working on your self-esteem will help you have a better self-image. A woman cannot feel sexy with a poor or negative body image. Remember that sex is done through the body, so if your "vehicle" is seen and is perceived negatively, there will be no pleasure on "the road."
- ▶ Medical side effects of pills and contraception: To feel safe and be responsible are basic requirements to relax and enjoy sex. When a woman does not feel protected from unwanted pregnancy, it will be very hard for her to relax and enjoy herself. Also, be aware of the side effects of the pills you are taking—and why you are taking them. The importance of shifting from pharmaceutical pills to a healthier way of treating problems, such as changing your diet, using herbs and supplements, increasing positive emotions, among other healthy options, currently stands out. Chapters 2 and 3, about health and emotions, may help you in developing better strategies. If you don't feel healthy, energetic, and strong, you probably won't feel sexy either—you won't enjoy sex!

As you may see, a lot of factors can impact sexual desire and sexual pleasure! These factors are all interconnected and work together against or in favor of your sexual happiness.

Part IV: The Pleasure Spectrum Model

I believe it is not just about having or not having pleasure—black or white—it is like most things, a range of different "intensities of pleasure" that fluctuates day by day according to our experiences and ways of thinking. Therefore, I have crafted a "spectrum of colors" to visualize the wide variety of pleasures, from no pleasure to beyond pleasure. I have named this spectrum of colors *The Pleasure Spectrum Model*. It displays the range and intensities of pleasures and its extremes by using colors. In this way, you can see the great variety of pleasures and locate yourself on the spectrum. It goes from plain white— anhedonia, no pleasure—to dark black—addiction, beyond pleasure.

White and black are the two extremes of the Pleasure Spectrum, representing around 20%, of the people suffering from anhedonia or addiction. The median—around 80% of the population—goes from mild to moderate pleasure, represented by light yellow and orange, to red—intense pleasures such as sexual pleasure. Intense pleasures, "the red zone," include not only sexual pleasure, but also emotional pleasures—like falling in love, as well as spiritual, and intellectual ones (I am experiencing intense pleasure in writing this book). Whatever it may be, intense pleasure evokes passion!

Let's now visualize the range of pleasures, from small ones to pleasures to intense ones. See the Pleasure Spectrum below to better visualize the wide range of pleasures:

The Pleasure Spectrum™

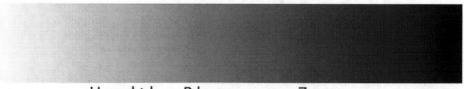

Anhedonia   Healthy Pleasures Zone   Addiction

Aleida Heinz, Ph.D., Copyright © 2019

The Pleasure Spectrum Model

Passion

When there is passion, pleasure intensifies, so passion intensifies pleasures, and intense pleasure will evoke more passion! I think they feed each other... In any case, intense pleasures and passion get along. The word "passion" is particularly used in the context of love and sexual pleasure, suggesting a deeper emotion. But social psychologist and associate professor at Loyola University Maryland, Theresa DiDonato, PhD, indicates that "passion includes sexual desire, but it's more than that."

Remember Sternberg's Types of Love in Chapter 3. A Complete/consummate type is characterized by having passion among its elements. Feeling intense pleasure for something will lead you to passion. We can say that we experience passion when we are experiencing intense pleasure for something or someone. Don't you want a passionate relationship? All of these start with the experience of happiness and pleasure. Passion is not only an element in the LOVEX Model, important for lovemaking as discussed in Chapter 3, but for keeping you learning, working, and *making love 365 times a year.* Benjamin Franklin once said: "If passion drives you, let reason hold the reins."

Can you see how happiness, desire, pleasure, and passion are interconnected? Isn't it fantastic? If you keep yourself navigating in the middle of the Pleasure Spectrum—having healthy pleasures—sometimes going from yellow to orange, and from orange to red, back and forth, and experiencing intense pleasures with passion, then your life could be more colorful—just be cautious about going too far in either direction, you may lose control.

Find meaning in your life; fight for what you want and what you like, find your passion in life, and in this way, you can enjoy intense pleasures while living with passion. *Making love 365 times a year* requires a certain degree of passion, so you can experience genuine, intense, and healthy sexual pleasure.

Navigating the Pleasure Zone

Think of yourself as a child on a playground. Have you ever seen a young, secure kid on a playground? They are not afraid to have fun! They are not worried about getting dirty or hurt. There are no problems, no restrictions, no fears. They just climb ladders, go down slides, try the monkey bars. They have not yet learned fear. Think about that. To "navigate in the pleasure zone" and enjoy sexual pleasure, you must learn to have no fear or concern for getting hurt, rejected, or judged. You cannot go into sex, especially lovemaking, with the expectation that you will feel pain, be judged, or get hurt—emotionally or physically. Instead, be like a child, exploring and testing your environment—and your partner. Learn about each other with no expectations!

Within sex, of course, there will be limits: your own limits and boundaries—the size, depth, colors, shapes, and boundaries of your 3rd Floor. These should be established before sexual activities, as we discussed it in Chapter 4. Like a parent will tell a kid, for instance, that they only have twenty minutes, or to stay away from the big kid's slide, before they play. The rules are established before the fun begins. As psychologist and author Hasselaar says, "everyone has the right to set their limits, and no one should ever cross those limits." This is fundamental to enjoying sex and surrendering freely to sexual pleasure.

Now think of the child who's afraid to play. They cling to their mother; they remember falling and getting hurt. They have doubts about themselves and others. These children have lots of stress, and what's more, they create stress for others. This is like a person in sexual distress. A child who is afraid to talk, to interact, might be called a "good boy" or a "good girl" by adults, but their fear is what drives them to be silent... This is not okay! Just like you may have been told not having good sex or experiencing sexual pleasure makes you a "good boy" or a "good girl," the child has been taught to be afraid, and so have you. To achieve sexual pleasure, you must unlearn these fears, any fear, and try new and better experiences again. It's not natural to be scared, awkward, or afraid of sex; it is learned.

Take a moment and observe how you act when you get into bed with your partner. Do you reach out to them? Play and tease? Or do you hide away, and snap "don't touch me?" These small actions may be what is leading to a lack of sexual pleasure. Your 3rd Floor is now your "sexual playground" for the "playing" with your partner. Act like it! Keep your body and soul naked. There should be no performance, just natural, pressure-free actions. Keep it simple. Keep it fun without holding back your feelings. To enjoy your sex life even more, and experience pleasure, it is important to have curiosity and feel inspired, energetic, and full of good vibes! Remember the importance of kipping good feelings as discussed in Chapter 3.

Once you experience sexual pleasure, the general pleasures you already enjoy will be enhanced! There are some things you can do to cultivate sexual pleasure. Through some effort, consistency, and dedication—and passion—you can achieve any goal. And if your goal right now is to increase sexual pleasure, follow these simple five steps. These steps have helped many couples in my practice:

1. Cultivate the desire to experience sexual pleasure and let go! In my experience, the root of low desire is the lack of pleasure. Desire is where it all begins. Tony Robbins said it best: "Desire is the first element of realization." You would not be reading this book if you did not desire more passion and pleasure in your love life! Focus on the desire of "desire-more" in order to experience and learn more. Resnick also says in *The Pleasure Zone* that "the first step in intensifying pleasure is learning to let go." Focus, relaxation, and awareness play a critical role in achieving sexual pleasure.

   Resnick advises that "the ability to enjoy pleasure is cumulative. If we hold back in any one of these eight core pleasures—primal pleasure, pain relief pleasure, elemental pleasures (laughter, play, movement, vocal expression), mental pleasures, emotional pleasures, sensual pleasures, sexual pleasures, and spiritual pleasures—every other pleasure will be limited by that restraint." Therefore, we need to be able to learn and enjoy pleasurable activities daily to fully experience sexual pleasure as well. In my experience, the pleasure of lovemaking is very close to spiritual pleasures, since, as suggested by Resnick, one aspect of spirituality "is to feel a part of something good," and that good thing is the deep connection that brings feelings of love when you are making love.

2. Only engage in sexual activities for pleasure and/or connection! NO other reasons! Even if you want to have a baby, it is best to be connected and enjoy the moment than to engage in sex mechanically—that's no fun at all! Little by little, you should be learning, or re-learning, how to find and feel pleasure. How do you reach out to that child who's afraid? By teaching them little by little that their fears are unfounded. You tell them that "having fun isn't bad!" Right? It is crucial to avoid at all costs falling into the bad habit of having sex by obligation, manipulation, or duty. According to DiDonato, "when people engage in sex out of a desire not to disappoint a partner, they don't experience any increase in sexual desire and the outcome is less relationship satisfaction." So, never ever have sex as a "job to do." But what if your partner is initiating?

Be affectionate in turn, if you don't feel like having sex, but don't push them away! If you want to experience sexual pleasure and *make love 365 times a year*, you must find ways to always enjoy it. Play in your playground, get dirty, and have fun!

Do you remember affection as discussed in Chapter 3? Well, now you and your partner can become masters in affection, so that you can shift any situation, including sexual approaches, into a calm, pleasant, and relaxing moment without the need to avoid, reject, offend, or withdraw from your partner. So, when any sexual initiation occurs, and one of you is not interested, simply be affectionate without even saying anything. If both of you apply give affection "as a code" of not having sex now, there will be no need to disconnect. In fact, by giving affection to shift the situation, you may receive affection back, which in turn may lead to an increase of spontaneous desire through anticipation with no expectation!

3. Enjoy small advances! Continually reinforce yourself that sex and pleasure are good for you. Create your small love habits to strengthen your sex life. Author William Jones says, "our life is a mass of habits," so you should make them good ones! You are learning something new, so enjoy it. Meg Selig, author of *Changepower!* and professor of counseling at St. Louis Community College at Florissant Valley, wisely advises: "make the process of changing pleasurable in itself. If you do, your brain will reward you by releasing some of that good "oh' feel-good" neurotransmitter dopamine, making you that much more motivated to change." Enjoy having pleasure in small skin to skin contacts, rubs, and caresses. Go slow and easy!

4. Make yourself AVAILABLE! Be present and let your partner know you are there ready for them. Do not hide, avoid, or get busy or distracted by multiple activities. One never finishes working or completing chores. Set aside the time to BE present and available for love. Get ready without demands or expectations; just be there, willing and available. By being mentally and physically available, fears disappear, and anticipation appears.

5. Think about CONNECTION! The only expectation is no expectation and connection! Remember that satisfaction depends, in part, on your expectations. If both of your expectations are to connect, you will both feel satisfied, even if you don't orgasm. This isn't about having an orgasm; it's about the pleasure of being close to each other and feeling connected. Higgins and Hirsch also found that women need sufficient stimulation— soft touch, good smells— as well as give-and-take of emotional intensity and the feeling of protection to experience sexual pleasure.

More Pleasure!

Think for a moment in your bedroom. Is it nice and comfy? This should be not only a safe place for you and your partner, but also a place that inspires lovemaking. So, everything in your master bedroom should be sexy and beautiful. Soft lighting, good-soft sheets, and some erotic art, including pictures of you two in happy moments. Keep it clean, private and quiet, remember, this is your "playground." Keep out of your bedroom: kids' toys and smells, bills, work, dirty laundry, and even family photographs—a picture of Great-Aunt Judy does not make for a sexy environment. Turn your bedroom into a provocative suite. Make it comfortable and welcoming for the two of to *make love 365 times a year...*

I ask the same question Higgins and Hirsch did in their study on pleasure, "can a genuine desire for sexual pleasure shape women readiness for sex, sexual exploration, initiation, and a more active and healthy sex life?"

I do think so!

Regardless of age, hormones, and background, any woman can learn to experience sexual pleasure, if she has a genuine desire and the mental condition for it. Experiencing sexual pleasure is essential to wanting more sex, enjoying it more, and being sexually happy. Great lovers don't think about performance and achieving orgasm. They think about connecting to their loved one, and what they can do before lovemaking to be outstanding. Beecham, from previous chapters, says: "great competitors know when and how to just play the game." The same is true for lovers: great lovers know when and how to just "playing the game" and *make love 365 times a year...*

"Nothing is as important as passion. No matter what
you want to do with your life, be passionate."
—Jon Bon Jovi

Part V: 7 Simple Suggestions & Recommended Sources

7 Simple Suggestions for Increasing Sexual Pleasure

1. What makes you happy? What about sexually happy? Take some time to meditate on the diverse activities that make you laugh and feel relaxed. It is crucial to be happy and cultivate happiness to better deal with everyday life. Nothing is worth it if you're unhappy, unhealthy, and crabby. I love this saying: "Do you work to live or live to work?" Think deeply about that and make a choice! Remember the 40% Solution: it is totally UP TO YOU be 40% happy by the THOUGHTS you choose to have, and by the ACTIONS you choose to engage in. Go LOVEX!

2. Use the Pleasure Spectrum to locate yourself in different moments in your life. Be aware when getting low in the spectrum—light yellow—to recharge your activities with enthusiasm, passion, and energy! Get passionate, but remember, not too little, not too much! Learn to maintain balance in your life, keep yourself and your love life navigating in the middle of the spectrum—between orange tones and reds. Find your passions in life, have a meaningful life, and *make love 365 times a year*!

3. Start by enjoying small and simple pleasures. Start by taking 10 minutes a day to go for a cup of tea or coffee and just enjoy it without thinking, reading, or being on your cell phone. No Internet, no talking; just enjoy your whole tea/coffee every day. I suggest you enjoy this simple activity always around the same time to make a good habit of relaxing and enjoying a little every day! Beside this, be sure to take some deep breaths throughout the day, to better deal with your responsibilities. Rest!

4. Practice deep French kissing every day or at least 3 to 4 times per week. Close your eyes, think nothing, and just be present. Learn to enjoy the moment—no worries, no fears, no expectations of any kind. Taste your partner's tongue, enjoy it; smell your partner's face with closed eyes, enjoy it; explore your partner's mouth, teeth, tongue, saliva while breathing slowly without any hurry, enjoy it. Get used to deep French

kissing; you will end up loving it! Hot kissing is a determinant to sexual pleasure!

5. NEVER EVER engage, agree, commit, perform, do, or have sexual activities without WANTING them, nor without PLEASURE! It is ok if you want to please your partner, but first, find ways to get into the mood before trying to please him or her. First, relax look for things to do that can help you feel happy and prepared for a sexual encounter. Go to your 2nd Floor first before jumping to the 3rd Floor, if you are not ready. Then, slowly, using your senses and becoming erotic (next chapter), start sensual and sexual touching. Go slow! Don't push, rush, or force yourself. Enjoy, so that you can experience pleasure in bed and increase the desire for more....

6. Use your best sexiest non-verbal communication to initiate and enhance your sexual encounters. Be romantic, slow, soft, sweet, loving, and expressive. Remember the importance of non-verbal communication and sexual expressions from Chapter 4. Remember that all pleasures can be intensified through making joyful sounds. Enjoy your new sexual mindset, have fantasies, move your body, *feel*, and don't think! Navigate your partner's body without expectations. Just be there—present in mind and body—to truly enjoy what you are doing!

7. If you feel a hole or emptiness inside of you and feel the need for help, go for it! Life is too short and beautiful to waste it. If you or your partner are unable to experience any pleasure in your daily life, seek help. Also, if you feel unable to control yourself, feeling out of control, either drinking or engaging in risky sex, etc., it is time to re-think your life and fix your pain. Enjoy pleasure without getting out of control. Seek help as soon as possible, so you can enjoy your life in a healthy way and have pleasure!

Don't fight your battles alone. There are plenty of professionals willing to help! You have only one life is one, live it to the max with love, happiness, pleasure, and passion! Live your life with LOVEX to *make love 365 times a year*!

Recommended Sources for Sex Secret #5

The How of Happiness: A Scientific Approach to Getting the Life you Want by Sonja Lyubomirsky, Ph.D.

The Pleasure Zone by Stella Resnick, Ph.D.

The 5 Second Rule by Mel Robin

Elite Minds by Dr. Stan Beecham

Changepower! 37 Secrets to Habit Change Success by Meg Selig

The Compass of Pleasure: How Our Brains Make Fatty Foods, Orgasm, Exercise, Marijuana, Generosity, Vodka, Learning, and Gambling Feel So Good by David J. Linden

Girls & Sex: Navigating the Complicated New Landscape by Peggy Orenstein

Why the thrill is gone: Scientists identify potential target for treating major system of depression. Study done by Goldman, Bruce https://med.stanford.edu/news/all-news/2012/07/why-the-thrill-is-gone-scientists-identify-potential-target-for-treating-major-system-of-depression.html Stanford Medicine, July 2012

Pleasure, Power, and Inequality: Incorporating Sexuality into Research on Contraceptive Use. Study done by Higgins, Jenny A., and Jennifer S. Hirsch. American Journal of Public Health October 2008

Why being in the mood is important for women. Study done by Kalmbach, David A https://www.anxiety.org/how-anxiety-depression-affect-sex-drive

The World Association for Sexual Health website: https://worldsexualhealth.net/declaration-on-sexual-pleasure/

SEX SECRET

6

CHAPTER 6

Eroticism

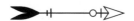

Eroticism is like a dance: one always leads the other.
—Milan Kundera

Part I: Understanding Eroticism

I can't agree more with famous song writer André Salvet that "the difference between eroticism and pornography is one of art." Yes! Eroticism is art, beauty, and the most sublime expression of sexual desire. Eroticism gives form, texture, and softness to the sexual approach, provoking the other, through the art of seduction, which turns the simple act of having sex and penetration into an exciting experience of infinite pleasure. We are now going to work on the fascinating art of "going there"—eroticism. This is the art of moving from one physical and mental state to another—neutral and closed to open and intense—that will allow you to enjoy your sexuality and let it go...with grace, enthusiasm, and elegance. I hope you will find these two chapters, Sex Secrets #6 and #7, fun and exciting!

Eroticism comes from the Greek word "Erys," meaning passionate love and sensual desire, and from the Greek mythology god "Eros." For the ancient Greeks, Eros was the god of love and the son of Aphrodite, represented as a young man with wings, a bow, and *arrows* of passion for shooting his victims with the fire of passionate love. This character is also known as "Cupid." His passion and lust have crafted eroticism—not the actual act of sex, but what precedes it.

Eroticism is related to sexuality and its projections by an exquisite exaltation, both physically and mentally, producing a deep interest in sex—it is what should precede the sexual act. The erotic feeling or emotional state is often mistakenly confused with fetishism (passion and desire for an object or body part), sexual compulsion (uncontrollable desire for sex), and even confused with pornography (sexually explicit entertainment for adults).

The best definition of eroticism that I found is: "Eroticism is a quality that houses sexual feelings and philosophical contemplation of the aesthetics of sexual desire." When you become erotic, you are entering the world of anticipation, sensuality, seduction, and desire. How fun! Usually, I can't wait to introduce eroticism and sensual techniques to couples who are ready for them. Unfortunately, most couples give up too fast and choose to stay in their comfort zone, holding back resentment and fears. As one of my favorite sayings goes: "it is easier to suffer than to take full responsibility for your life and personal growth."

It is not until a couple reaches healthy levels of interaction, empathy, compassion, trust, positive feelings and thoughts, and intimacy—a solid 2nd Floor—by having eliminated resentment, destructive habits, and strengthened their connection, that they can enter the sphere of eroticism and the art of great sex. If it was, otherwise, it would be a total disaster! Exploring your erotic self should be fun, easy, and exiting—an adventure within yourself—but you must have put some work into the previous chapters first. Usually, "you have to get worse before you can get better." By confronting your old mindset and beliefs, getting healthier, having positive feelings, being able to express yourself, and being able to experience pleasure, you are now ready to explore your erotic self. This is awesome!!

Now, how important is eroticism for *making love 365 times a year*? Very important! That is one of the questions couples in a good place ask me, and my answer is: Eroticism is an imperative element to keep the flame of passion alive. But these couples also always ask me: how can passion be kept alive? By increasing EROTICISM, as well as putting your partner FIRST, and paying ATTENTION to them, you can maintain passion through time. Therefore, eroticism and passion go hand-in-hand to give more flavor and life—"sabor, ritmo y vida"—to your sex life. Both elements play a crucial role to fully enjoy *making love 365 times a year*, in a fun, durable way...

Let's see through Case #6 how eroticism plays an important role in sexuality, and why it is a key component for passionate love life.

Case #6: Julie & Mark and Felicia & John

Once again, we will be looking at two cases that are very different but have the same problem. Our first couple is Julie and Mark. Julie is 31 years old, and Mark is 32, they've been married for one year and have no kids. They knew each other for nine months before they got married. The second couple is Felicia and John; she is 36, and he is 41. They have been married 11 years and have two kids, ages 10 and 5.

In both cases, partners come from different cultures—cross-cultural couples. This can often lead to problems with eroticism because different cultures perceive or use eroticism in different ways. In both cases, we see a lack of eroticism and can understand why this is an important part of their sex life.

Julie and Mark came to see me together. Julie explained, "I just want to improve our relationship. We have some problems and want to solve them."

I asked her to elaborate on their problems.

"I have a hard time enjoying our sex life," Julie said. "I feel restrained. I've never felt restrained in my past relationships. Those all ended because we didn't have the same goals or the same things in common. But I've never had problems with sex."

Julie explained that they had fun together and liked to travel. When it came to sex, she enjoyed it but rarely had an orgasm. Mark seemed exasperated.

"I don't understand what's going on," Mark huffed. Her lack of enjoyment meant he had withdrawn his sexual advances.

Recently, they had been avoiding sex even though they liked it and had the desire. Both still masturbated when they were apart. Even when I talked to them separately, there was no hidden resentment or communication issues. They were both healthy and happy.

"I want him when we are apart..." Julie said. "But I freeze up when we are together!"

This situation had created friction in their relationship.

As we continued to talk, I found out that when Mark wanted sex, he asked her for it in a very direct, mechanical, and unsophisticated manner. "Do you want sex?" he'd spring on her.

"It's like he's asking me what's for dinner? or Do you want coffee?" Julie complained. "There is never any pre-foreplay involved with Mark." Yes, and I agreed that there was not "art" in setting up the moment for sexual intimacy.

"The moment I start touching him, he just directly asks if I want to have sex," Julie continued when I spoke with her alone. "Sex now feels too mechanical. I don't feel pulled or driven..."

Now we know, eroticism was what they needed. The affection was there; he seemed very kind to each other, but Mark was attempting to jump right from little affection into sex. He was missing some steps!

Felicia, a member of the second couple, came to see me alone, as John refused to join her.

"I don't know what to do," Felicia began. "A long time ago we struggled with communication, but we fixed that. Now we enjoy our sweet love, but in the past few years, it hasn't been fun. John just wants to get right to sex. He will turn to me and goes "hey honey, on top?" and nothing else!"

John was just asking for sex with a preamble, and only occasionally. Felicia had the same frustration and needs as Julie.

"I feel like I'm riding a mechanical bull," Felicia complained. "He pulls it out, I climb on, and that's it. There is no heat!"

Felicia could get herself going, but to do all the work herself every time meant that sex was not be fun anymore. And if sex is not fun, you will not desire it or seek it out!

Many times, couples will become too comfortable with one another, losing the seduction and craving that go along with eroticism. You have grown too familiar! And while affection and love remain intact, there is no longer any need to impress, conquer, provoke, seduce, and attract one another.

Be aware that affection and love are healthy and necessary but are not enough to sustain a passionate love life. Pure affectionate love cannot be all there is! You need to seduce your partner to provoke them every day to avoid robotlike approaches to sex.

In fact, many couples feel ridiculous when doing this, becoming apathetic to the idea of seduction and eroticism, and losing lots of fun and pleasure, as we may observe in these cases.

"Oh, seducing him is silly," Felicia argued at first. "I've gained some weight and don't look the same. I don't feel sexy to be seduce John. Besides, he knows how I look like." Then, she thought again... "Maybe! That would work... sounds fun!"

See Julie and Mark Lovemaking Wheels:

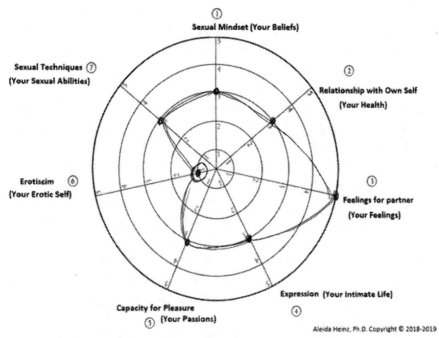

Julie's Lovemaking Wheel. Wheel #11

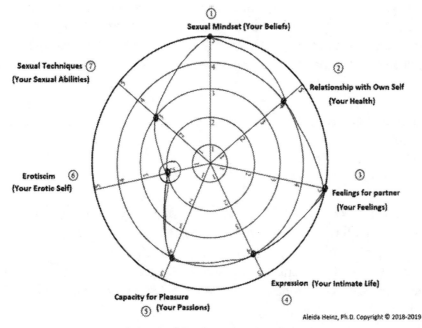

Mark's Lovemaking Wheel. Wheel #12

In both cases, these couples were missing eroticism. They had to be taught to play the game again—and not just occasionally, but all the time! You can be affectionate but also erotic, to sustain passion. Both elements—affection and eroticism—are very different, but highly important and essential to sustaining a heathy, non-conflictive sex life. And I will tell you why…

Katehakis, from Chapter 2, has defined eroticism as "vital energy to create and connect…the intention to arouse sexual desires in oneself and the other." Eroticism precedes sexual desire and sexual acts! Remember, to me, the root of the lack of desire is the lack of sexual pleasure, so how can you have pleasure if it is not fun and provocative to go there? It is "the dance" that triggers desire, and strong desire leads to sexual attempts, and if it is pleasurable, then feelings of satisfaction will come up, leading to more desire—wanting and liking it even more.

Mexican poet and 1990 Nobel Prize winner, Octavio Paz, recognized as one of the major Latin American writers of the 20th century said: "Eroticism is exclusively human; it is sexuality socialized and transfigured by the imagination and the will of man. The first note that differentiates eroticism from sexuality is the infinite number of ways in which it manifests itself, in all epochs and in all lands." Let's explore this in more depth…

Morin in *The Erotic Mind*—from previous chapters—describes an erotic equation that explains eroticism and demonstrates its importance to sex. His formula or equation is very simple: Attraction + Obstacles = Excitement. Then, Morin goes on to list the "four cornerstones of eroticism"—giving shape to his formula:

1. Longing and Anticipation
2. Prohibitions
3. Searching for Power
4. Overcoming Ambivalence

Longing is defined by having a strong, persistent desire or craving, especially for something unattainable or distant. As Morin wrote, "part of being human is the ability to picture in your mind something or someone you desire but don't have or isn't there." It is about craving something or someone you already had and miss (the past). On the other hand, anticipation is the advance realization of something to come (the future).

These two elements shape your dance, or erotic moves, toward that person you desire—make that person be your partner; that is, keep your partner in mind. You can imagine and vividly fantasize what will happen next if you dance, and so give yourself a short try of "dancing" together. According to Morin, "longing and anticipation are variations on the same theme; both draw energy from the gap between desire and the reality of the moment." This is just fascinating!

You may realize now that eroticism is not sex, and it has nothing to do with pornography; it is the intention to have sex or make love. You reach out with your "dance" to create sexual feelings. Eroticism is, then, "the dance" you play before and during explicit sexual acts to slowly wrap the desired person and seduce them until you possess them. This is an art that needs to be cultivated with time and practice. In our youth, hormones lead sexual acts; at more mature ages, eroticism should lead sexual acts—including lovemaking—no hormones, just sexual and erotic minds…

Eroticism: The Stairway to Sexual Pleasure

My personal and professional experience has led me to understand eroticism as a "powerful connecting element" that connects one situation to another, escalating its intensity toward sexual pleasure—leading or not to sexual acts. So, I have crafted a "stairway," which I have called *Eroticism: The Stairway to Sexual Pleasure*, to illustrate and explain eroticism as a connecting element, in a simple, visual way.

Affection, or at least appreciation, is the foundation that supports the stairway—*Eroticism: The Stairway to Sexual Pleasure*—where you start building up, step by step, the context to, then, sexually enjoy and experience sexual pleasure. All the process of "going up the stairway" should happen in a sublime, subtle and delicate way—and, at the same time, exciting and provocative.

Let's see the stairway that I have crafted: *Eroticism: The Stairway to Sexual Pleasure*.

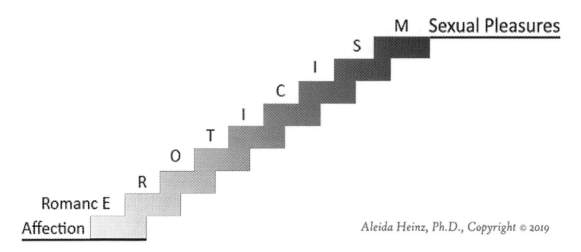

Eroticism: The Stairs to Sexual Pleasure

What a fantastic way of climbing and increasing sexual tension, creating a context where you and your partner can freely experience sexual pleasure. By using the stairway—eroticism—you and your partner can go from your daily routine to a place of lust, passion, and desire. Imagine the base of the stairway in yellow—appreciation, affection. Then, as you go up, colors start changing, like more intense yellow to orange, and then color pink—romance. Gradually colors intensify until they become red to then dark red—sexual pleasure, "the red zone."

Let's recall the Three-Floor House from Chapter 4. Eroticism is the best way— "the stairway"—to go up to your 3rd Floor: the mental and physical space to experience sexual pleasure. So, now imagine that you are in your living room sharing as a family. Then, imagine that you want to have sex—to go to your 3rd Floor—but you don't know how to initiate or if your partner will go with you. What would you do? How do you go from one "space" to another? Or, in other words, how do you go from the 1st Floor to the 3rd Floor? Do you just jump? Jumping will be very hard, leading to frustration, and no pleasure. But what about if you use the stairs? Wouldn't it be easier?

That's precisely my point. If you want to move from a non-sexual to a sexual state or space, use the stairs, do not jump! The stairs are eroticism—*Eroticism:*

The Stairway to Sexual Pleasure. You need a "stairway" in your relationship—in your Three-Floor House—so you don't have to "jump" and suffer. Robotlike or mechanical sex feels as if you were jumping without any previous preparation, making the whole experience annoying, complicated, and frustrating, as in the case of Julie and Mark. Quickies are different; you are already "there!" When you are in an erotic mental state—3rd Floor—that will allow you to enjoy sex anytime, anywhere, and with no time, then, you can enjoy quickies! But quickies should be the exception, not the rule in your love life.

Building together, as a couple, a solid and reliable "stairway to go there" can become a relaxing activity; but you need to learn more about eroticism first. Do you see how fun and easy it can be to *make love 365 times a year*? But you need to start building your stairway in your Three-Floor House now! It's never too late for eroticism in your life…Let's do it.

Please observe the Three-Floor House but now with the addition of *Eroticism: The Stairway to Sexual Pleasure.* A complete, passionate relationship needs eroticism to sustain its passion throughout time.

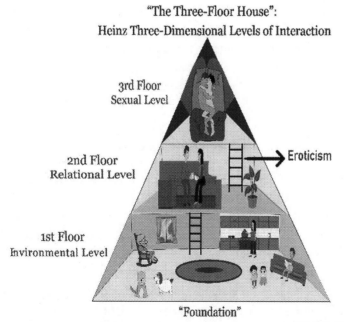

"The Three-Floor House":
Heinz Three-Dimensional Levels of Interaction

3rd Floor
Sexual Level

2nd Floor
Relational Level

→ Eroticism

1st Floor
Invironmental Level

"Foundation"

Aleida Heinz, Ph.D. Copyright © 2019

The Three-Floor House Model plus Eroticism

You will climb the stairway more often because now it is fun and exciting. That means you and your partner may engage more frequently in sexual activities because you have learned about eroticism and are using it to change your mental state in order to enjoy the moment and experiencing sexual pleasure. Even if you are not in a committed relationship, it is still a great tool to go from a nice friendly time to a hot sexual moment. There are many differences between human sexual activities and animal sexual performance, and one of these differences is eroticism. It works for all humans in diverse ways and styles. Find yours!

We are born with a wonderful capacity to imagine, fantasize, recreate, and improve our sexuality, beyond the simple act of penetration and procreation. All this capacity for sexual thought, fantasies, and emotions reaches a mental sphere of intellectual influence, which is translated as eroticism: a mental/emotional state primarily belonging only to us, the human species. I have realized that it is easy to become lazy when you feel too comfortable in a long-term relationship, so neither of you makes any effort to seduce the other.

And once a couple, like Julie and Mark, stops trying to "climb the stairway," they begin to extinguish the passion between them, losing the curiosity and the interest to have sex. Likewise, they are also wasting one of the greatest treasures we have as sexual beings: our capacity to be erotic and seduce one another... When the desire is gone, and is fire was extinguished, what you are probably missing is eroticism in your love life, as well as romance. So, let's become erotic!

Part II: Becoming Erotic

The first step towards becoming erotic is your attitude. Then, practice and try different behaviors, manners, and ways to express yourself, in which you feel confident and sexy. Go slowly, be patient with yourself, and maintain a positive attitude toward revealing your erotic self; step by step you will enjoy the journey—climbing the stairway. Remember, it is about "the way" you are choosing to "get there." The results vary, according to your attitude and effort.

Remember this: you need to take time if you want to make love. That means, prepare the way... The transition from being "mom or dad" or "worker or housekeeper" to being lovers takes time. Not taking enough time for such a transition from one role to another, but instead rushing, pressing, or jumping to sex, may only bring frustrations. Use your stairway—*Eroticism: The Stairway to Sexual Pleasure*—for the transitioning of roles and interactions.

Attempting to seduce and provoke your partner will induce more desire to "climb the stairway." This process is all about imagination, creativity, curiosity, exploration, playfulness, fantasy, and, most importantly, your willingness to "get there." When you enjoy more, you want more, and will connect more. That's the goal of eroticism. Becoming erotic is, then, becoming fully alive, aware of all your senses and using them. One of these senses is touch. Touch, as we learned in Chapter 4, is essential, especially when becoming erotic. But touching should now be more sensual and slower, intended to provoke and awake sexual feelings, not just to exchange affection. Also, movements and actions play a huge role when becoming erotic. Do not neglect taste, smell, sight, and sound, as they are key to the "game of seduction." Use your senses to create sexual expression; this will lead to the creation of your own unique erotic language.

Katehakis has found that "touching and hugging" are the main promoters of erotic feelings. There is always a good time to hug and touch your partner... Create moments; don't wait for something to happen; seize those opportunities. When you are preparing yourself and your partner for lovemaking, you are erotic. When becoming erotic, you start moving slowly—like a snake—across your stairway, stepping into your stairs while slowly changing your mood and actions. This is fascinating to me! It is a world of imagination and anticipation... It is an art! As Czechoslovakian author and critic Milan Kundera said best, "eroticism is like a dance: one always leads the other."

For me and many of my colleagues, exploring your erotic self is essential for sustaining a passionate relationship. It's the way to bring everything else together and "go playing" with your partner. Although animals have their own techniques to attract a mate, they are not erotic. It is disheartening to know that there is not much research on eroticism itself. But what scientists have found is that people enjoy sexual activities more when there is eroticism.

When you become erotic, you are more inclusive. You play with another human, your partner, so you include them in your erotic game. Inclusiveness is great for relationships! When you exclude your partner, you are avoiding, denying, neglecting, or rejecting them, as if your partner were a "roommate." When you are inclusive, you are inviting your partner to play with you and share pleasurable experiences—together.

Eroticism in Your Life

Become erotic outside the bedroom; it's about your home having a touch of eroticism to remind you of your erotic nature. It can even be a new way of living. Relax and incorporate the following tasks into your routine and enjoy it!

▶ Create and be creative
▶ Be uncertain about life's outcomes, enjoy surprises
▶ Fantasize more
▶ Get out of your daily life, be curious and observant

These four tasks may not be easy at first, but they are necessary to go beyond your comfort zone and explore your erotic self. Your state of mind should be more inclusive with your partner and freer to play...

You should constantly be provoking and seducing your partner. You can reach out, even when you're apart, by texting or calling your partner with sensual ideas: "remember last night," "I'm still thinking of you," "your name is etched into my skin," etc. Once you start thinking of them in an erotic way, it will be much easier! And, when you are together, you should always be touching, hearing, and smelling one another. Keep the eroticism going—climbing the stairway every day!

Six habits of highly erotic people have been identified, and they closely mirror the work we have been doing in this book. While not a scientific study, it is a great reminder of all the important parts that make up our sexuality and our erotic selves. The six habits of erotic people are:

1. Savoring life: Pleasure and eroticism go hand-in-hand. That's why we have already learned that pleasure, and discovering pleasures in everyday life, needs to come before eroticism. In my view, first, you develop your full capacity to experience pleasure, and then work on your erotic self. Knowing how to relax and have pleasure helps you be more erotic and then to enjoy sexual pleasure.

   Eroticism is about imagination and cultivation of pleasure. You don't want just to be surviving; you want to be living! So, forget from now on the robotlike sex, performances, and sex acts loaded with expectations. Pleasure and eroticism are the opposite of all of that. If you integrate eroticism into your life, the rest will follow. It is all about having better sex, and *making love 365 times a year...*so, savor your life!

2. **Being confident and having self-belief:** One of the sexiest attributes a person can have is self-confidence! If you feel sexy, you can feel erotic. If you have insecurities, how can you work on your eroticism? Remember Chapter 2, when we worked on your body and building confidence in yourself. Without confidence, you hardly can be erotic. Instead, you will constantly be doubting yourself.

   This also ties into getting rid of resentment and anger, as we discussed in Chapter 3. For eroticism to exist, you must clean up your feelings towards your partner. If you are clean from all resentment, then you have the freedom "to go playing" with your partner. You two can handle your relationship in a more sophisticated way where eroticism can thrive.

3. **Talking until there's nothing left to say:** Talk before, during, and after sex! There's nothing wrong with occasionally enjoying the silence, but overall, you and your partner need to communicate and express your passion! In Chapter 4, we talked about how to use expression to create sexual intimacy. You need to talk and non-verbally express yourself! Don't focus on complaining, but on sharing information and desires. What did you like best about lovemaking? What turns you on? What sexual fantasy did you have today? Just hearing the words can be highly erotic, especially if you enhance them with your senses. There is nothing more enticing than sharing and expressing enjoyment when you *make love 365 times a year...*

4. **Cultivating curiosity about strangers and strange things:** Part of the connectivity you need to have with your partner comes from exploring weird things. Remember the example from Chapter 4, where we thought about how a child is free at a playground to explore because they feel safe in their mother's love. It's the same in your relationship. You need to feel stable to be free to explore and cultivate eroticism. Feel free to try things that might seem "weird" at first.

Always work together as accomplices, confidants…you don't want to get bored! Creativity and novelty are about thinking and trying new things, instead of doing the same thing over and over. Curiosity cannot coexist with shame and fear. This inquisitiveness is essential to eroticism. But of course, you already have built trust and intimacy, first—Chapter 4.

5.   Challenging prejudices and discovering commonalities: You and your partner shouldn't be tied to just one thing. Like in Chapter 1, your sexual mindset must be open to new ideas and facts about sexuality. Do not live surrounded by fear, myths, and false sexual morality; the things you were taught as a child. Erotic people challenge these prejudices. Rethink what you were taught as a child and see what hampers your sexuality and eroticism. If you spend your life sexually repressed, you will explode! That is not healthy nor erotic…

6.   Cultivating wanting: Nothing is more erotic than anticipating pleasure and sharing it with your partner. Savor that feeling of "if I don't have you now, I'll die" or "I want you now," with a tender and maddening look. Like we talked about, you need to build tension with one another throughout the day. Fight to *make love 365 times a year* with passion and eroticism! Start provoking one another. Make it fun and hot! Today is your tomorrow…

Forms of Erotic Expression

There is nothing like visual arts and sensual music to awaken and cultivate your erotic self. Erotic art, which has nothing to do with pornography, has been for centuries the best way to cultivate eroticism. Much of this art comes from ancient Greece and Rome, with amazing erotic sculptures and paintings.

But look beyond just the ancients—today we can find great erotic art surrounding us. Erotic artist Victor Newsome said, "the erotic aspect of my art is not pornography but magic, animation, and evocation. My figuration makes no references to figurative art or pop art but arises simply because I view this world from inside a human figure and tend to feel an affinity with things which appear human." Erotic paintings and sculptures are in abundance everywhere around us, from ancient times to modern times, presented in many forms. Pedro and I love them, and we are always looking for some fun and beautiful erotic art to decorate our home. These are some samples of erotic art:

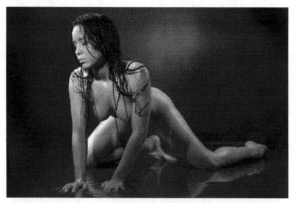

EROTIC ART

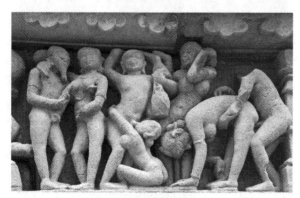

EROTIC ART

The same is true for movies and plays. Movies are another great way to keep eroticism in your life—and in your mind. Again, I am not referring to porn, but movies that made you think about lovemaking, passion, great sex, and help you focus on sensuality. For instance, some French movies can be very erotic, like the *Emmanuelle* series—sophisticated and sensual. Also, *The Piano,* an erotic movie from the 90s. Why do you think 50 Shades of Gray was so popular? Because it is erotic. Movies like this one may not be erotic for some people—especially for men—but by watching them together, it can awaken your erotic selves with imagination and fantasy. Once your partner sees how turned on you are, they will appreciate the erotic aspects of any movie...

Erotic literature may help your erotic self to wake if you prefer to read. Fantasy, stories, and tales, as well as comics, are also fun ways to explore eroticism. I found music highly important to let go of the erotic imagination. Singers like Sade and Barry White are, to me, probably among the best-known erotic singers I know. A musical genre like *Bossa Nova*—my favorite music—could eroticize any environment. But the choice is yours! Explore different ways of expressing eroticism and awaken your "sexy you," either through art, movies, plays, music, or other forms of expression. The idea is to find what is erotic for you and your partner.

From the time of the ancient Greeks to the modern day, eroticism has been a huge world to explore. There are even classes and workshops you can take to learn how to make your life more erotic! As you dive in and learn how to share this world with your partner, you will learn what turns you on and what turns on your partner. Eroticism should be part of yourself: how you look at, talk to, move with, and seduce one another. You can learn erotic movements from sexy people like Marilyn Moore, Sofia Loren, Brad Pitt, Motahari, Cleopatra, Antonio Banderas, to mention a few...from the past and from the present. Also, how you dress, and eat, walk, and look at one another can be erotic. It is about the *attitude* you adopt to increase desire and sexual tension.

You can be erotic in public, too, in a healthy way. Dress up when you go out, look sexy for yourself and your partner. Don't dress as you do at home; make the time you spend together special. Visit erotic places where there is low lights, good food, and good wine. A good dinner out can be erotic and produce the sexual tension you are looking for—depends on your attitude.

All of this should build up to "I WANT YOU."

In the same way, make your bedroom an erotic place for you; this will keep your sexual environment provocative—your 3rd Floor. Also, if you like, you can have some erotic art as you develop your sexy setting and intimate space. For instance, in my bedroom, I keep pictures of Pedro and I kissing...to refresh those moments! A TV in the bedroom it is okay as long as you watch it together—and wisely. Your TV can be used as a tool for connection; that is, for the two of you share different kinds of experiences through movies. Use your private TV for your erotic movies and make sure it's turned off if you aren't actively watching it together. The rest of your house might not be as erotic, but your bedroom and suite bathroom should be!

Expressing Your Erotic Self

Expressing yourself is important for sustaining a passionate relationship—Chapter 4. Now is the time to express your erotic self. You can do that in different ways by, for instance, creating an erotic language that only the two of you will know. Now that you know how to become more erotic and have a healthier romantic relationship. Expressing your erotic self in healthy ways has some great benefits for you and your partner:

▶ It shifts yours emotional and mental state, which acts on the nervous system, driving you back to sexual desire and pleasure, and to reconnect to your partner.

▶ It enhances yours and your partner's senses: touch, sight, smell, taste, hearing. This can be done through erotic art, erotic literature, erotic music, and every action that may lead to sensual delight—I will explore the senses in Part III.

▶ It improves your imagination and sexual fantasies. Don't avoid them but enjoy them. Through thoughts, creativity, and imagination, erotic feelings may positively impact your love life to the extent of experiencing transcendental lovemaking.

▶ It sensitizes yourself and your partner physically and psychologically for sexual expression. Women, especially, need to be ready, through a positive state of mind, feeling wanted and comfortable, to have and enjoy sex.

Passionate behavior with an erotic mind is the key to an outstanding sex life, which will truly nurture the whole relationship. There is a strong connection between sex, the brain, and eroticism. Eroticism lives within the brain and will travel throughout your body through your senses, making you and your partner more sensual. As Argentine sexologist, Ezequiel Lopez Peralta, says, "sex is limited while eroticism is infinite." I share with Peralta the suggestion to open our structures and become more flexible, thus learning more in order to become happier beings, free and able to express our desires—always in healthy ways.

Katehakis suggests "start inviting eroticism with an open-minded, open-hearted intention, ritual or meditation right this moment. Trusting yourself is key to the expression of your eroticism and will be made evident when you challenge yourself to be honest about your sexual arousal." Don't hesitate, it is part of who you are! Be erotic to recreate the spice in your relationship and to *make love 365 times a year*—with passion!

Part III: Becoming Sensual

What makes a sensual person? What is it to be sensual? Is it essential for connection and lovemaking? YES! It is crucial. Sensuality is awareness, sensing, and perceiving your environment and the people around you. It is crucial to understand the importance of awareness and being sensitive to feel and incite your partner. Sensuality is about all your *senses* "being awake." A state of being sensual means that you are sensing—*feeling*. When you use all your senses, you are also awakening the senses of your partner. You are sensual when you are fully aware of your surroundings and fully aware of your partner. We are sensual beings; we just need to awaken our senses to feel. How then could you feel your partner?

There are many different definitions of sensuality, meanings, and interpretations. By joining all the descriptions, I can undoubtedly say that sensuality is a state of high mental clarity that allows us to feel the body and perceive the environment in a sensitive, vibrant, and relaxing way. By perceiving the environment in this way, we evoke a mystical, exotic, and even romantic experience where we become "sensual." When you become sensual— conscious and fully alive—you are using all your senses that, according to Peralta, are "the gateway to eroticism."

Today, most people are too busy with the demands of their lives that little by little, without realizing it, begin to lose what makes them happy. The birds singing, the smell of flowers, the sound of rain and all the little fundamental things no longer seem relevant. Life goes by without them even having tasted it! They look like dead…and, in times of crisis, their dullness worsens. A quote by John Lennon that best describes this sad reality is: "Life is what happens while you're busy making other plans." Those "other plans" usually don't include spending time with your partner, having deep conversations, or making love. Too often, those plans include working, business, watching the news, the Internet, taking care of your family or community, or other duties.

These "other plans" can dominate your life and dull your senses, so you become insensitive to life and your partner. Remember that "lose what you don't use!" Therefore, it is possible that you, not only become blind to your feelings and desires and your partner's but also your sensuality—unable to feel. I agree with Huffington, from Chapter 1, that "when we integrate death into our daily lives...it transforms how we live; it transforms everything because it brings perspective into everything." Death is a certainty that will make us appreciate every day so much more. You aren't dead, but you are going to be. So, don't waste your life by stressing, depressing, or becoming bitter; live it with passion and pleasure; your senses are there for you to experience life—and your loved one. Then you will live your life to its fullest!

Awakening Your Senses

TIME TO WAKE UP! Wake up your senses to retain your passionate sex life! You cannot be passionate if you are asleep. Start by focusing on today, the here and now, right now! People who are not aware of their senses are unable to perceive the moment. The good news is that you can "train" yourself to be aware and fully present. When awareness of life is translated into your love life, you become capable of experiencing a whole new world of sensation to truly make love—using your five senses—and of maintaining aliveness in your love life.

Remember, one of the habits of highly erotic people is that they savor their lives. Savoring life means to taste, smell, observe, hear, and feel your surroundings. When you savor your love life, you are feeling, smelling, tasting, seeing, and hearing your partner. Indeed, it is through your senses that you become erotic, and at the same time, when you are erotic, you become sensual, feeling each other. In such a way, eroticism and sensuality are intertwined, nurturing each other to experience intense sexual pleasure.

Part of the training to awake your senses is perceiving everything around you through your senses. The way you experience the world is through your perception channels, but everyone emphasizes different channels. As part of my training in Neuro-Linguistic Programming (NLP) long ago, I learned to stay quiet for a while to sharpen my ears and hear the soft and different sounds in the distance. It is truly fascinating! Also, I was trained to feel different textures without seeing them and observe the world around me closely, among other things. For instance, I love to stand in the woods and try to distinguish far-off sounds, to see in the distance, and to distinguish different smells. This is called conscious awareness exercise. You can also train yourself in such a way—we are all sensual beings. First focus on only one sense at a time, eventually, you should be able to focus on a crowded block in New York City and find a bird amongst the cacophony of noise.

It is fantastic everything that happens around us without realizing it. We really miss a lot!

In NLP, you learn that some people are strongly visual, while some have strong taste or auditory senses. In general, it has been found that women are predominantly auditory, and men are more visual, as I mentioned before. But everyone is different! Learn what your main channels are and then share this with your partner. And most importantly, note all of them, use and develop them all. As far as we know, the five sensory channels of perceptions—your five senses—are:

1. Visual/Sight Channel—what you see
2. Auditory/Sound Channel—what you hear
3. Kinesthetic/Touch Channel—what you feel
4. Gustatory/Taste Channel—what you taste
5. Olfactory/Smell Channel—what you smell

You can discover your predominant channel—based on how you usually express yourself—and find out your partner's as well to understand each other better. Pay attention to your use of words as well as your partner's. Of course, we use all our senses, but we will naturally gravitate towards one or possibly two.

Visual people are more apt to use phrases like "I see," "let's see," "watch this," "I have a vision," etc. Auditory people usually say, "I hear you," "sounds good," "that sounds like," "I'm listening," etc. Kinesthetic people usually use words such as "I feel," "I have the sensation," "I touched," etc. More unusual are gustatory people who talk about the taste and spice of life as well as olfactory people who talk about smells, like "doesn't smell good to me," and what smells they remember.

The book The Perfume is about a man who worked so hard at sense of smell to the point of becoming a perfume expert. The Perfume shows an excellent example of training a sense, in this case, the sense of smell—the most powerful sense. You can also train your sense of smell to be a great lover—but do it without killing your partner or anyone else! It is very important to be aware of this particular sense because: it's not love at first sight; it is love at first smell!

The Olfactory System

Some studies show that the olfactory system is the most powerful and primitive of all. You will pick up smells faster than you will fully see someone. When you first meet a potential partner, you smell them before you even see them! Moreover, the olfactory system, like no other system, is highly successful at triggering emotions and memories, bringing unexpected powerful responses almost instantaneously. This system is so powerful that it can influence our mood, for good or bad, because it is part of the limbic system of the brain, an area associated with memory and feeling.

Jordan Gaines Lewis, PhD, postdoctoral researcher at Penn State College of Medicine, has done extensive research on the olfactory system. Gaines has found that the olfactory system, "more than any other sense, triggers more vivid emotional memories and is better at inducing that feeling of 'being brought back in time' than images." That means that smell is the most powerful sense, even stronger than vision. How is this possible? Gaines explains the amazing connection between smelling and feelings. Smells are fast detected by the olfactory bulb and then run back through the brain. The olfactory bulb (in our noses) has direct connections to the amygdala and hippocampus in the brain—areas strongly involved in emotion and memory. Gaines pointed out that "interestingly, visual, auditory (sound), and tactile (touch) information do not pass through these brain areas."

In fact, many recent studies show a strong correlation between smell, memory, and emotional intensity. So not only do you remember, but you may feel the same emotions you did back then. Memory also triggers and elevates brain activity, elevating the emotional potency of the evoked memory, bringing great visual vividness as well. This holds for positive and negative emotions as well, not just for one or the other. Pay attention to what triggers positive memories and, thus, positive emotions. Likewise, notice what triggers the negative. Gaines states that "smells can also be potent triggers of negative emotions, particularly in individuals with posttraumatic stress disorder (PTSD)." So, you might re-experience the overwhelming feelings through smells and odors, making you avoid situations or places where these scents can be.

Moreover, a study done by Herz and Von Clef found that people rated an identical odor as more pleasant when it was presented with a positive label rather than a negative label. Therefore, positive labels—your perception and beliefs of something—have also a great impact on how you feel about something.

Now, my point is, with all this information, can you see how positive, and especially negative past sexual experiences can influence your love life? Smells, odors, and scents automatically recall past experiences—making you and your partner re-experience them. If past experiences were negative, they might be overwhelming for you, triggering unpleasant feelings, thus messing up your entire love life!

Smells and Your Love Life

Are you aware of these powerful reactions in yourself? Probably not! Usually no one is! Especially if you started your sex life at a very young age or had unwanted sex early on in life. In fact, most young people have negative sex experiences due to a lack of self-knowledge and proper positive sex education, as we mentioned in earlier chapters. Remember the Netherlands studies, where it was found that in the USA, most young female teens have negative first sexual experiences. Therefore, bad memories probably formed.

In addition to this fact, sex has, in general, a negative label, making the situation even worse! Remember the Herz and Von Clef study that found that, people rate identical odor as more pleasant when it was presented with a positive label rather than a negative label. Consequently, if a person had unpleasant sexual experiences (smells and odors unconsciously tied to the experience) plus negative labels (such as sex is wrong, dangerous, dirty, etc.), what do you think will happen in the adult life of this person when they want to have sex with a committed partner? All the negative memories stored in the olfactory system will suddenly come up. It will be a total disaster, don't you think?

Smells in your bedroom can have the same effect; the smells of sweat, cum, vaginal fluids, saliva, or even a certain deodorant or perfume can trigger and bring back vivid bad memories that will cause a person to pull away unconsciously—rejecting the negative experience of the past, and not their partner. Sex odors are usually similar, triggering pleasant or very unpleasant memories, and thus unpleasant feelings, according to their labels and the person's past experiences.

It is crucial to understand that, as Gaines points out, "individuals can have widely divergent emotional responses to scenes that are identical in composition." What does this mean? Some scents don't come from the same place but can have the same chemical composition. A crucial one, in this case, is semen. Semen coming from different men can have mostly the same chemical composition. So, this can trigger huge negative emotions and memories of past negative sexual experiences, if they were harrowing enough to cause such reactions.

If you had terrible or traumatic sexual experiences in the past, probably smells from those experiences have been stored in your brain. Therefore, future sexual encounters might have very similar smells—triggering unpleasant memories—making you feel avoidant and confused (even if you are now with a lovely different partner in a different place on earth). These specific smells will still bring back negative memories and emotions. You will begin to block out and avoid sex because you are re-experiencing trauma from the past.

Resetting the Olfactory Memory

Negative memories may be back there waiting to be triggered by smells! So now you need to consciously REPLACE them! It is beyond working to have a positive sexual mindset, a positive attitude toward sex, good intentions, love, or sexual desire; it is about targeting at the most primitive of all system, your olfactory system. This primitive system stores, deep down in your brain, unpleasant memories registered through the sense of smell. A way to modified or "refresh" those negative memories is by consciously—intentionally—storing new and refreshing positive memories from the present—resetting and updating your olfactory system. Therefore, you must get fully involved in new, positive, and pleasant sexual situations and attach the odors to these experiences. It is not an easy task, but probably the most effective way to overcome the frustration of not being able to enjoy your sex life.

Now you need to believe but also behave (remember the two Bs in Chapter 1), take ACTION and go for positive sexual experiences, feelings, and sensations, making use of all your senses, especially the olfactory one. So, SMELL your partner to build up new different and positive memories, that eventually will be stored for the future. In the present, you are building your future... Storing new positive experiences is one of the many reasons why it is so essential to awakening your senses, especially when you are making love. According to Gaines, "unlike other animals, humans have evolved to rely more on our sense of vision, but their sense of smell may be more important than you think." Making love provides a unique opportunity to explore our senses.

Smell your current partner more consciously. Only then can you create different feelings and memories. So much desire and passion are now available to you! So, create positive memories to *make love 365 times a year* for the rest of your life! Find pleasure in smelling your partner. The goal here is to have positive memories from pleasant smells and then re-experience them over and over. You then may be turned on just from smelling your partner, so great sex will be around the corner! You can now experience sex freely with no trauma.

Sensuality in the Bedroom

What about in bed? Now translate all you have learned about sensuality and your senses to your bedroom. Image yourself smelling, tasting, hearing, and feeling your partner, and your partner also "savors" you. Provocative, isn't it?

What a magnificent gift is to have full conscious awareness of your senses when you are making love—to truly make love. To feel, smell, taste, and hear each other...to be able to listen to those little expressions of pleasure, the sound of your flows, the soft sighs and whispers in your ears...the taste of your kisses, of the saliva, the feel of each other's tongues, the breath, the skin, the smell, the sheets... And then, to feel each other's hot bodies, the sweat, the smell of sex, and the taste of your flows, your wet genitals, the texture of the nipples, and each small part of each one's body. This experience only can happen if both of you are aware of the moment, only focusing on one another and perceiving through all your senses. It is pure sensuality, precisely where passion, desire, sexual pleasure, and satisfaction reside.

When you are making love, train your ear to hear sounds of pleasure from your partner while noticing the smell of your partner's cum—if your partner is a man. You need to be very tuned into your partner; this is critical. Be present and make your senses present as well, for new experiences and new ways to respond and discover what turns you on and makes you passionate.

It is not until now that the perfect moment to start *making love 365 times a year* has arrived! The moment to sexually express so much desire and passion! The art of eroticism and sensuality have made you ready to play and seduce your partner, to possess one another entirely...ecstasy may enter in the equation, for even more "playing." Sex coach and psychologist Amor Antunez suggests varying the shared sexual sensations and experiences by inserting changes in, for example, the schedule, the location, and even the furniture, to intensify the sensual—and erotic—experience or playing.

Professional tasters are expert on tasting the different molecules in food, wine, beer, etc. You can enhance your senses to become an expert on tasting your partner's body, and that's exactly what makes you a great lover. *Making love 365 times a year* will be so fun, so easy, so exciting, and so "natural," so you will repeat the experience over and over, making it your "new normal"—what a fabulous love habit!

Become an expert on your partner—and in yourself. Wake up, wake up your partner, and wake up your all senses. As Gaines says, "I hope your life is full of good smells, good feels, and good memories!"

Part IV: Seduction

Although for many the term seduction may have a negative connotation, it is really the opposite. Seduction is very positive if you understand its meaning well, and you intend to attract your partner for good. Seduction is commonly defined as "the process of deliberately enticing a person to engage in a relationship, to lead astray, as from duty, rectitude, or the like; to corrupt, to persuade or induce to engage in sexual behavior." A legal definition of seduction also goes like this: the act by which a man entices a woman to have "unlawful sexual relations" with him using persuasions, solicitations, promises, or bribes without the use of "physical force" or violence. What?

If you notice, both definitions, like many others, have assigned to the act of seduction negative interpretations, referring to seduction as unlawful sexual relations, corrupt, etc., where usually men are the evil and the antagonists... now think, with such definitions, who would dare to seduce?! These outdated concepts of seduction, far from helping us get closer to our partners, slow us down and paralyze us, making us believe that seducing is a bad and perverse act and, preventing us from even seducing our own partner!

Now, think again!

Seduction goes beyond the intention to engage in sexual intercourse; it is much more than that! It is about attempting to attract someone—in this case, your partner—pursuing them so they will be with you. It's related to allurement, enticement, temptation, appeal, attraction, charm, enchantment, conquering, and power. It is about the inclusion and closeness to one another that every couple needs. I believe we require all these attributes as part of our lovemaking equation. Seduction is closely related to sexual activities, but it is not necessarily about that. Remember, it is about attraction and closeness. It is part of the "stairway to sexual pleasure," helping to build tension. Therefore, it is highly important to constantly seduce your partner and have your partner seduce you as well. It is part of being erotic and part of the "game of love."

Seduction can also be related to business, home life, shopping—anything! It is the act of enchantment, of convincing people to do what you think is good. It is most obvious in politics! Author of *The Art of Seduction*, Robert Greene says, "no political campaign works without seduction." The 19th century is really when seduction entered politics—people were seduced on masse by political candidates. Now, marketing and advertisements use seduction as well, both sexual and non-sexual, to convince you to purchase their products. Greene calls today's seduction "a war of penetration." This is a theme of psychology, the penetration of your mind. Therefore, any time you watch an ad, that company is trying to seduce you into using their product. Greene continues by saying that "nothing will give you more power than the power of seduction."

In fact, seduction is all about pure psychology and strategies You need to become your own marketing expert, using seduction to get what you want—your partner! Here, you particularly want to focus on seducing your loved ones.

Seducing Your Partner

Founder of The American Fertility Association and author of *Shameless*, Pamela Madsen, tells us that "seduction is all about savoring. If you rush things, you can miss the best part. Living a happy, juicy life means extending the pleasure, and we can do that with learning how to enjoy and practice seduction and anticipation. Savor everything and use the joy of seduction as a path to pleasure."

The whole idea is that you see your partner not as your sibling or roommate, but as someone you must conquer and whom you want to attract in order to *make love 365 times a year...* Always recall that when you are in any long-term relationship, it is easy to get too comfortable and lazy. Initially, your love life may have LOVEX—see Chapter 3—but as time passes, you begin to see your partner/spouse as "family," taking passion, lust, and, probably, sex out of the equation—preventing you from seducing one another. This "familiarity" is what kills passion.

Felicia, from our case study, thought the idea of seducing her husband was silly, just as if I had suggested she seduce her roommate. This is an epidemic in the United States as we discussed before, the longer a couple is together, the more sexless they become. You need to see your partner as your lover; it doesn't matter how long you have been together, or how old you are. Lovers must seduce each other. So, start enchanting your partner now! Remember *Eroticism: The Stairway to Sexual Pleasure*; seduction is an exciting "step" of the stairway that builds up your way, to lead you in a smooth, slow, sexy, and fun way. Again, seduction is not sex; it is, as Kitty Cavalier of the School of Cheek and Charm says, "the thrill of the desire itself. It is the game that is played as the desire comes closer, and closer, and closer, and being able to maintain that tension of wanting for a long, long time."

Use your erotic skills and your sensuality to seduce your partner to slowly "go playing," with own love codes either for "going there" or "staying here." If you want your partner, you need to pursue them. Don't just roll over and say, "it's time for sex," "I want to have sex," or "you never initiate..." like our case couples, going from 0 to 100—from the 1st to 3rd Floor—without climbing the stairway! It is like driving a sports car from 1st gear to 5th in a minute! Poor car...just in a rush, like telling them to take out the trash now!

You need to seduce your partner, and conquer and attract them, so you aren't imposing upon them. The awareness of your partner is essential for lovemaking. If you internalize the importance of this, you both will be able to *make love 365 times a year* in pleasurable ways. So, pay attention to your partner as you did in the beginning. Believe that you must make them want you.

While seduction can be used for personal gain, this is not our aim. Just because it can be used to manipulate, doesn't necessarily mean seduction in and of itself is wrong. Throughout history, there are examples of men using seduction for their gains. But here we are using seduction to build upon your loving, passionate, and lasting relationship.

Seduction Strategies

According to Greene, the first great seducer for love was Cleopatra. She is the first known female seducer in history and is well-known for her introduction of seduction into politics. She used her beauty, enchantment, sensuality, appeal, behavior, and actions to conquer Julius Caesar. She used her seduction to conquer. Greene refers to this type of seduction as the "female strategy." The strategy is about being visual and uses behavior, actions, and sensual movement to enchant the person you are after. After Cleopatra, men began to impose power upon others through seduction as well. It is a more psychological way to gain power, using language and enthralling behaviors.

Two of the first sexual seducers were Don Juan and Casanova. Is it any wonder they are Spanish and Italian? We've talked about Italians and their thirst for life. This isn't a new idea! Especially when compared to Anglo-Saxon and Germanic historical figures, those from the Mediterranean are always seen as more seductive. Research backs this idea up; the happiest couples come from Italy! A large part of this is because of their passion for life, and one another, is very high. Couples from Italy, Hispanic and Portuguese countries kiss frequently and have sex more often than couples from other countries, as I mentioned in earlier chapters. Does this have something to do with seduction? Of course, it does!

Greene calls Casanova's approach the "male strategy" for seduction. It is more verbal than the female strategy. We don't know exactly why the Mediterranean is best at this, but they seductively use their language. In these cultures, men have worked on their language skills to seduce their female partners better. And at the same time, females have worked on their body movements to seduce men. Therefore, I suggest that combining female and male strategies—seductive vocabulary plus sexy body language—will be the ultimate form to seduce and conquer your partner, regardless of gender or age!

The reason this works so well is that you are seducing people through their *senses*. So, instead of thinking only about your senses, you should be thinking about your partner's senses as well. Men are usually seduced through the visual; they find images and pictures more enticing. So, women learn to use a visual strategy when seducing a male partner. For example, red nails, dress in red, sexy clothes to call the attention of a male partner.

Meanwhile, women are more auditory, so men learn to use words to seduce their female partners—as the saying I mention before, women have a clitoris in their ears! Is this a set-in-stone-works-for-everyone rule? No! But science backs up the tradition, showing that in most cases this is true. When you first begin seducing someone, these strategies are the best starting point. In your own relationship, you need to learn what senses turn your partner on most and play to those. I'm not saying that a man needs to be a bandit like Casanova, or that a woman needs to look like a super-model to seduce their partner. But you do need to have self-confidence and use that aspect of yourself to entice your partner. Women may explore their femininity in the way they dress, lingerie if desired, soft manners, etc., and at the same time, can use their masculine side to reach out as well.

In the same way, men may explore their masculinity, being secure, self-confident, supportive, reliable, etc., and at the same time, explore the feminine side by concentrating on feelings, and using soft and sexy expressions. There is nothing more seductive and provocative than the awareness of the conscious exchanges of masculine and feminine roles between each other within the relationship.

Learning to Seduce

According to Greene, seduction always has two elements we must be aware of:

First is YOU—you need to be a fountain of seduction. Do this by knowing yourself and what you find sexy about you, as we discussed in Chapter 2. Know your strengths—mental and physical—and use them to attract your partner.

Second is YOUR TARGET—who do you want to seduce? In this case, it is your partner you want. You need to know how best to seduce your partner, what they will find sexiest. Learn how to be the seducer they will want.

Greene, in *The Art of Seduction,* has identified nine types of seducers. Pick one or the ones you prefer to enhance your skills as a lover. You can also combine all these nine types and make your own type! The nine types are:

1. The Siren: Based on the male fantasy. Mostly used by women. Here you become highly sensual and confident; your physical appearance is your greatest power. You need to use your body to seduce, not just with your beauty, but sensual body movements. According to Greene, Cleopatra and Aphrodite are great examples.
2. The Rake: Based on the female fantasy. Mostly used by men. Here you always make your partner feel wanted and desirable. You need to be very verbal, open you heart, and be sensitive. Be intense, passionate and attentive to your partner. A good example of this is Don Juan—and Pedro...
3. The Ideal Lover: Male and female fantasy. Used by men and women. Here you need to become an ideal person for your partner. Be very adaptable, and please your partner. Observe and find out what your partner needs, then do it! According to Greene, Casanova is the best example.
4. The Dandy: They are free lovers with a free spirit. Use your attitude to attract your partner. You need to combine the male and the female strategies depending on the situation; so be soft, romantic, and

passionate at the same time. Valentino is the best example, according to Greene.

5. The Natural: Childish and innocent. Here you need to be curious, innocence, naive, and softness to seduce your partner. Think of a child-like wondering.

6. The Coquette: Mostly used by women to confuse men. Here you delay satisfaction to make a game of anticipation for your partner. You need to be very erotic, independent and sensual. Give and take, be unpredictable. Build up tension to seduce your partner. According to Greene, Josephine, the first wife of Napoleon, is the best example.

7. The Charmer: You need to be highly creative, offers pleasurable and novel activities to seduce your partner. Focus only on your partner. Everything must be about your partner.

8. Charismatic: This type of seducer is seen most in politics.

9. The Star: The all-around perfect fantasy. Most movie stars and musicians use this type of seduction, where their life doesn't even seem real. There is no fighting, no drama, no problems, no stress; all in life is just fun and pleasure, seduction and enchantment.

When crafting your seduction style, only think about what your partner would like. Just have fun. You only want to seduce your partner in a good way—not to manipulate.

Eroticism, Seduction and Sensuality

It doesn't matter if we are seducing a man or a woman; the visual and auditory channels of perception are very powerful for both genders and work well when conquering and seducing someone. But don't neglect the rest! Just start being aware of these two senses, and then the rest will follow—and always remember your powerful sense of smell... So, be sure to always smell pleasant to your partner (especially breath and genitals). Lots of turn-offs occur just by the simple interference of bad smells or unpleasant essences. According to the HealthPrep Staff, "stronger body odor is a sign of a complication or high glucose levels." Having a healthy lifestyle (Chapter 2) will help you emit more pleasant smells.

Food can be used as seductive tool; with a fancy meal, vision (the way you and the environment look), hearing (soft music and sexy words), smelling (your essences and delicious food), and taste (each other's lips, the wine, and the food) can all trigger desire by seducing each other's senses...

Being erotic and sensual to seduce your partner is a healthy and fun way to persuade them to be next to you, and "going up" using your stairway to enjoy your 3rd Floor. You and your partner want to have a beautiful, active sex life and *make love 365 times a year,* so go ahead and seduce your partner every day! That is why you are together! Seduction, sensuality, and eroticism are human ways to create a provocative context to make love with passion.

> "Eroticism is invention, endless variation, but sex is always the same."
> —Octavio Paz

Part V: 7 Simple Suggestions & Recommended Sources

7 Simple Suggestions for Becoming Erotic and Sensual

1. Resnick, in *The Heart of Desire,* says, "erotica is women's porn." So, grab your partner and watch or read romantic and erotic movies or literature; it is for everyone, especially if you're a female or have a female partner. Visual stimulation through erotic movies or images builds desire. Sexually explicit presentations can also be very erotic; pick some to watch together to create sexual fantasies, romantic crushes, and lusty feelings.

   Learn more about eroticism and what it means for you and to your partner. Allow yourself to explore and incorporate erotic ways of doing things, like behaviors, mannerisms, movements, ways to talk, to see each other, to dress, even to eat! Try, little by little, different ways to express your erotic self. Don't be shy! Confidence is the foundation of being erotic.

2. Make yourself and your partner experience pleasurable sensations. Slowly taste delicious food, using your whole palate. Take a fruit you love and slowly eat it with your eyes closed, but eat it by tasting it, smelling it and sucking it—take your time. Also, wear something soft like silk, and feel it on your skin. Grab a deep tissue rub and rub your back, legs,

arms, etc., and feel the different textures. Sleep naked in soft silky bed sheets and enjoy the sensations on your skin…

3. Sit quietly, eyes closed. Relax and imagine yourself and your partner; your faces, the colors on your clothes, the things you are doing together—make the image get hotter and more intense, little by little. Be in that imaginary moment; feel and see yourself interacting happily and sensually with your loved one. Visualize the scene you want to live with your partner, bring the scene closer to you, bright, light, beautiful, and exciting. Enjoy your visualization and repeat it every time you can! Grab your partner's hand while doing it. Feel your partner's hands. Do it while visualizing and without visualizing, too! Enjoy!

4. Go to nature, close your eyes, and hear all the small sounds from those far away to those near you. Stay there, just listening to all kinds of sounds like birds, the wind, the rain, and far-off noises, too, like cars or people talking. Train your ears! While hearing, try to also smell the different odors near you, even your own.

5. Play with your partner and get dirty! A fun activity is to lie down in the bed naked, then, by taking turns, smell, taste, lick, suck, bite, and kiss your partner's body, starting at the face and ending at the toes. To enhance the experience, you may add textures and flavors such as feathers, whipped cream, chocolate, strawberries, ice cream, ice, or and any other thing you like! Try and be creative…surprise your partner! I am not talking about having intercourse and orgasm. It is about dirty hot erotic play. Of course, orgasm and everything else can happen consequently… they are always welcome!

6. Train your ear to hear small sounds of pleasure from your partner, notice the smell of your partner's cum, give a massage to your partner, touch them, and enjoy being touched. Get in tune with your partner. Smell your partner at different times throughout the day, especially when having sex, at night and when you first wake up in the morning, especially when doing your Pretzel Time. What's their smell like before and after sex?

7. Smell and taste each other's genitals, not with the intention to orgasm, but to associate your partner's sex organs with good feelings of pleasure. Do it as much as you can so that you both get used to each other's scents and odors. Do it regularly, like when you are in bed, taking a shower, or making love. Enjoy it!

Recommended Sources for Sex Secret #6

Perfume: The Alchemy of Scent by Jean-Claude Ellena

The Art of Seduction by Robert Greene

The Erotic Mind: Unlocking the Inner Sources of Passion and Fulfillment by Jack Morin, Ph.D.

Mirror of Intimacy by Alexandrea Katehakis, Ph.D.

Shameless by Pamela Madsen

The Heart of Desire by Stella Resnick, Ph.D.

Smells Ring Bells: How Smells Triggers Memories and Emotions by Jordan Gaines Lewis, Ph.D.

El Erotismo Infinito by Ezequiel Lopez Peralta (Spanish)

Sexo con Cinco by Amor Antunez (Spanish)

SEX SECRET

CHAPTER 7

Sexual Techniques

➤—⊪——◦⊩▷

The only unnatural sex act is that which you cannot perform.
—Alfred Kinsey

Part I: The Mechanics of Sex

F inally! Our last chapter, Sex Secret #7! I find this is the most sought-after Sex Secret, searched for by many couples, and, interestingly, searched for by those in "sexless relationships" (or, as I say, non-sexual relationships) wanting to "fix" their love lives. In fact, when I talk to people in dysfunctional relationships, the first fix they ask for is usually the mechanics of sex, but in my opinion, it should be the last thing they go for; they are missing the best thing about being in a relationship: the connection.

Please do not get me wrong; the mechanics of sex is as important as the other Sex Secrets, it is the last, but not least, Sex Secret which all lovers must know it. The point is, many couples try to move from dysfunctional systems directly to "fixing" the sex they don't have, without first working on any of the underlying problems in their relationship. Jumping straight into the mechanics of sex will make you lose the beauty of intimacy, passion, and eroticism among other elements. In that way, things between you and your partner can worsen as you try to improve your relationship by learning *only* about sex.

The LOVEX model (Chapter 3) isn't only about sex; it is also about love, lust, intimacy, and passion coming together to help you *make love 365 times a year.* Knowing how genitals work will not connect you to your partner, and, according to my experience, it is *not* the first thing to work. Focusing only on sex is one of the reasons why many relationships fail. These couples take an expensive trip to the Bahamas to "fix" what's wrong by hoping to have sex. You may have good intentions, but that's not enough, you need to do some previous work to "re-pair" yourselves again.

It is not until you have strengthened other aspects of your relationship that learning and applying sexual techniques can be beneficial and enjoyable. For instance, you may learn better oral sex techniques. So what? Learning a sex position won't stop your fighting, bad feelings, or resentment. But now you feel like you've tried to fix the relationship and you've failed. But really, you've simply treated the symptoms, not the illness. Only by combining the knowledge from all the earlier chapters can you work on techniques. You need to keep your entire Lovemaking Wheel big and round!

Now, in our car analogy, the mechanics of sex are "the motor of your car." We know everything about using the car; this is what makes the car run. It's important not just to have a motor, but to know basic car mechanics, like "where to put the gas." Back in Venezuela, gas attendants always put the gas in the car for you. When I moved to America, the first time I had to pump my own gas, I was a mess—I even got gasoline on my clothes! It sounds crazy, but if you've never done something, even something basic, you need to have some amount of learning and direction—in this case, some direction about the mechanics of the female and male bodies.

The world of sex is extremely broad and has many different layers that you need to keep discovering and working on together. In this chapter, we will explore a bit about positions, oral sex, porn, role-playing, anal sex, kinky sex, open relationships, and how sex works—which is fun, but, again, it will not "fix" your relationship by itself. On the other hand, not knowing sexual techniques or the mechanics of sex can also ruin your entire sex life. How can you experience mind-boggling, pleasurable great sex if you don't know what you are doing?

Let's see our last case—Case #7—for how a lack of sexual knowledge might prevent a couple from having happy sex life.

Case #7: Aliyah & Adam

This is an unusual case about a couple, Aliyah and Adam, who were frustrated about their poor sexual skills. This case is the best representation, I found, of the impact of ignorance of the basics of sexual functioning on relationships. Aliyah and Adam were a young couple that came to see me because they were exasperated by not being able to "have sex."

As I usually do in my practice, I went through the entire process—all the chapters we've discussed—with them, and they scored well in each of the six sections. Their Lovemaking Wheel was nice and round, except for one aspect—sexual technique! In the end, their wheel looked like a giant pizza with a slice taken out.

Aliyah and Adam were virgins with no previous sexual experiences when they met, and were now in their late 20's, married for three years with no kids. Not only were they virgins, but they were also one another's first everything—first kiss, first date, first sex. Much like I would be baffled about how to fix my TV, they had no idea how sex worked. They were having a hard time when trying to have sex and please each other.

When they first sat down, I asked about their current sex life. Adam spoke first: "I can cum, but alone; we have a great relationship. I am attracted to her, and she is attracted to me. We are just trying to figure it out..."

Aliyah continued, "our problem is that I am always initiating to try sex, and he is always rejecting me."

"I am not rejecting you," Adam interrupted. "I am avoiding the situation... I mean sex..."

But why, for what reason?

"This topic—sex—is too complicated," Adam explained. "I have been trying to make her have orgasms, but I do not know what to do or how to do it. We are open but do not know how."

"I don't know what to do either," Aliyah said.

I asked them about their previous experiences and learned there was none. They aren't into porn and only had very basic sex ed at school. They had no idea about orgasms.

"How do I know if I have had an orgasm?" Aliyah asked. Neither of them could tell if she had ever come.

For the past six months, they had tried to learn about sex over the Internet but were just confused about what they had read. They tried watching porn but didn't like it and didn't find it instructional. I spoke to them each individually and found they were not holding any resentment or ill feelings. Their problem was unique, as most couples have an array of issues, and this couple only had one and very specific.

"We have too much access to each other," Adam explained.

I had to ask him what that meant.

"We get naked, lay in bed. I kiss her, but I do not know how to do oral sex or if I should put my finger in her. She is just lying there. I could do anything, but I do not know what to do. I do not feel confident."

"I cannot do oral sex either...it is complicated," Aliyah said. "When I touch his penis, it just goes soft. I guess we are too aware of what we are doing. Sex is just an act and we do not know what to do with our own body parts. And now I am too tired to try anymore. I do not know how we are going to have a baby because he is afraid of hurting me when he tries to be inside of me."

They were both quiet for a moment before Aliyah continued.

"I am losing my desire to try again and have sex."

Let's observe the Lovemaking Wheels of this couple, which I consider unique and very interesting. See Aliyah and Adam's Lovemaking Wheels below and notice how low they both scored on sexual techniques; their wheels are almost identical with only one area of remarkable problems for both:

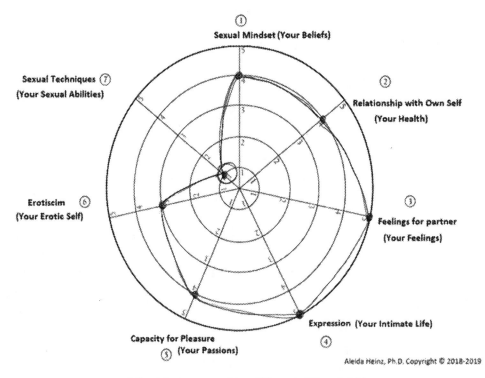

Aliyah's Lovemaking Wheel. Wheel #13

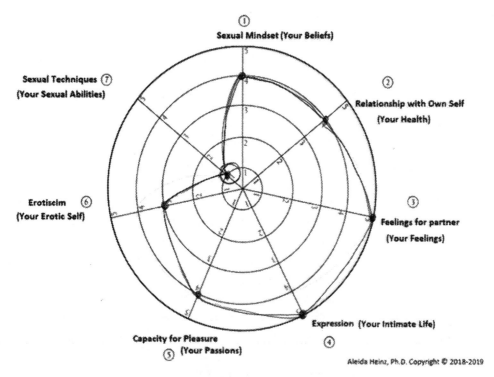

Adam's Lovemaking Wheel. Wheel #14

Fortunately, Aliyah and Adam had a very good relationship with no resentment, despite their sexual issue. Both enjoyed a healthy lifestyle and positive sexual mindsets, various pleasures, and even some eroticism, but were totally naïve and unknowledgeable about sexuality. It was beautiful to help them and see the joy in their faces after learning about each other's bodies, and genitals and their functioning, allowing them to finally experience intense sexual pleasure and connection. After some time learning about the topic and practicing together, they both reported some sexual satisfaction and even that they were expecting a baby.

Remember, this chapter is about sexual techniques and the mechanics of sex, but you cannot enjoy them if you don't already have a good foundation together. Learning about the mechanics of sex starts by learning a little bit about sexual anatomy to be able to be "playing" with it… Some people may worry that some of these techniques or ideas may hurt their relationship. They will not if you have first built intimacy and can talk about them openly and agree. For example, if you decide to add sex toys, it is because you both agree to it and know that these sex toys are just helpers to enhance your sex life. The mechanics remain the same as your goals—to be connected.

Part II: The ABC's of Sex

Once we figured out that they were missing the mechanics of sex, Aliyah and Adam became a fun couple to help. But there are still many couples, more than you can imagine, who are lacking the basic knowledge of sexual anatomy. So, let's review it, because it is something you need to know to become a great lover. I'm not discussing sexual reproduction at all; it's about what you need to know to practice amazing sex, and of course, to *make love 365 times a year*!

It can be tempting to use slang terms when discussing private parts. The problem with these words—such as pussy, cunt, dick, etc.—is that they can mean different things to different people. Is the pussy just the vagina, or the whole vulva for you? Does the clit factor in? Some people include the scrotum when talking about a dick. By using the appropriate words, you can better communicate what you want. However, in your privacy—3rd Floor—it will be fine, as long as you both know what you are referring to. The use of dirty talk and sexy expressions is part of your erotic equation.

Basic Sexual Anatomy—Female

First and foremost, you must know that the key to satisfaction, and the main sexual organ for females—besides the brain—is the clitoris. Clitoris comes from the Greek word Kleitoris or Kleis, meaning "a key," and from the German word der Kitzler, meaning "the key or the Klitoris." The clitoris is the key to female sexual pleasure and orgasm.

Second, you need to know that the female sexual organ has two parts, the internal (vagina) and external (vulva). In essence, it is as if women had two sexual organs, one for reproduction and the other for pleasure. So, it is crucial to differentiate them, vagina and vulva, to know what you are doing.

The Vagina

The vagina is the internal sex organ—the most popular and searched by heterosexual males, but less appealing. You will only find and see the vaginal opening (the hole). Then, inside is the vaginal channel, with its walls and floor—like having a "house" with walls and a floor to support the house. The penis enters through the vaginal channel—a muscular tube, around 9 to 10 cm long. Inside, you will find the vagina walls, starting with the vaginal opening, the G-spot, the Bartholin glands, the inside extension of the clitoris, and the cervix.

The G-spot, still in debate, can be a way to orgasm and female ejaculation, in some cases—squirting. The vagina, and by extension the G-spot, is connected to the clitoris. Notice that only around 20% of women can experience orgasm from intercourse alone, and the vast majority don't. Of course, most women enjoy penis-in-vagina intercourse, but without the stimulation of the clitoris, orgasm might not happen for most women.

After childbirth, some women lose sensation in their vagina, particularly around the perineum, located between the vagina and the anus. This area can be very sensitive, especially if it was torn or cut during delivery. But this does not mean anything; the capacity to orgasm and have pleasure is there and always will be regardless of childbirth—vaginal birth or cesarean section.

The primally functions of the vagina are:

1. To be a channel for the elimination of menstrual fluids.
2. To receive and enjoy the penis (or pleasant objects, like a dildo) during sexual intercourse and hold and pass sperm.
3. To provide lubrication through the Bartholin glands, ubicated in the vaginal opening.
4. To serve as the birth canal to deliver a baby.

For centuries the focus of having heterosexual sex has been on pleasing men and to please their penises—penis-centered mentality—where the penis is the king and protagonist of almost all sexual encounters. The penis-centered mindset is the main reason for the emphasis on vaginal sex because the penis finds pleasure in it—the penis likes wet and tight holes! But the fact is, penis-in-vagina intercourse is usually pleasurable but isn't enough for female orgasm and satisfaction!

Blood flow increases towards the woman's genitals, which in turn causes the vaginal wall and labia to swell. Like men, women also need a blood supply to be aroused, but the difference is that women need more than double the blood to engorge the whole pelvic floor than males need to get the penis erect. This is one of the main reasons why women need more time—at least 15-20 minutes of continuing stimulation—to be fully aroused. So, BE PATIENT!

When we "update" our sex life, we realize the importance of the vulva, and the clitoris, in heterosexual and lesbian relationships. So, there should be no more protagonists—instead, knowledge of one another's bodies for mutual pleasure.

The Vulva

The vulva is the external part, the one you can see and must focus on. The clitoris—the clit—belongs to the vulva, and its ONLY function is to provide pleasure and orgasm—nothing else. The clitoris—the central organ for female pleasure—is often ignored and misunderstood in many societies. So, please, if you are female or have a female partner, your primary focus should be on the vulva, not the vagina.

See how crucial the vulva is?

The vulva includes everything you can see: the Venus mound, the clitoris, the labia majora and labia minora, the urethral opening (urination, and in some cases the female ejaculation), the vaginal opening, and the perineum.

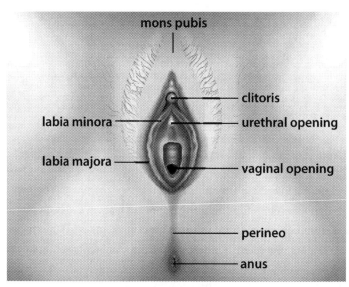

The Vulva

The clitoris is NOT a little button, as we were told, and many believe. Instead, it's a very big and large sexual organ, mostly internal, with only a small part of it on the outside. The clitoris is about 7 to 9 centimeters long—almost as long as the vaginal tube! It gets erect as well when aroused, but this growth is a little difficult to notice, due to its small size.

Around 18 different parts of the clitoris have been identified, including 8,000 nerve endings—twice as much as a man's penis, with only 4,000 nerve endings—and there are over 15,000 nerve endings throughout the whole pelvic area. The clitoris is connected to every part of a woman's sexual organ, including the vagina. It is interesting to note that it seems that a woman who has had her clitoris removed cannot orgasm. But a woman can get pregnant and have a baby without experiencing orgasm.

The clitoris is the only organ in the entire female body dedicated solely to pleasure. Think of it this way: whoever you think created the female body, gave women a clitoris for pure enjoyment and orgasms. Why? It makes no sense to create such a fantastic and powerful organ not to use it. There must be an essential reason, which has nothing to do with procreation, to have created this organ. As far as I know, it is to give us mental health through pleasure. It's a gift!

The primally and only function of the clitoris is: pleasure

Later we will talk a bit about orgasm, but for now, please enjoy the vulva or your partner's vulva if it's your case.

Basic Sexual Anatomy—Male

I think male sexual anatomy is much simpler—which doesn't mean better! Like women, men also are capable of multiple orgasms, but they need training themselves accomplish it. Also, many men enjoy having the testes played with, and some find the perineum, between the scrotum and anus, highly sensitive. Male nipples can also bring a man sexual pleasure. I have met some men who prefer nipple play even more than their female partner! But, for men, the primary sexual organ is also the most prominent one—the penis.

The Penis

An organ that is flexible and soft when not aroused, and large and hard when aroused: the penis. A penis engorges with enough blood flow, so good blood supply is the main thing for a penis! As I mentioned in Chapter 2, ED is often caused by blood flow problems to the penis. So, working out, exercises, and healthy eating can improve the overall health of a penis.

The penis is men's main sex organ—besides the brain—and the most sensitive area to sexual pleasure, which doesn't mean that they have no other sexually vulnerable regions in the body. Contrary to women, men's sex organ—the penis—has multiple functions: sex, urination, ejaculation, procreation, and pleasure.

The penis is comprised of the head, the urethral opening, the neck, and the body. Inside the penis are the urethra channel, the two corpus cavernosum that are filled with blood, and the corpus spongiosum. Like the vagina, the penis is made of embryonic tissue that can expand with blood flow. Behind the penis is the scrotum, where the two testicles are. As I mentioned before, the penis has 4,000 nerve endings.

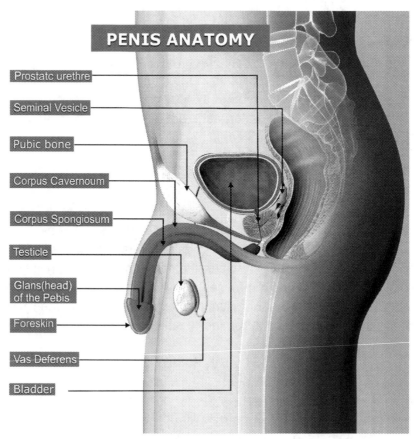

The Penis

Knowledge in Action!

After some time, or in many cases, after many years of sexual inactivity with a partner, you may be confused about what is going on with your body when having sex again. For many people, it is difficult to understand how the body works when having sex. In masturbation, of course, you go through a cycle of response, but we usually don't pay attention to it.

Now that you are ready to take action—or more action—and *make love 365 times a year,* it is important that you and your partner know how your bodies work and respond to sexual activities.

Stimulus and Response

First, researchers and scholars agree that to have a response; there must be a stimulus. But if the stimulus isn't enough, it not the right one or is done incorrectly; a response will not occur, as simple as that. So, there must be a stimulus, and second, there must be a response. Knowing what sexually stimulates your partner is essential. Conversations about what turns you on are necessary. There is not a "right" or "proper" way to be turned on, or to turn your partner on—the stimulus—every person is unique, so you need to know yours and share it with your partner; so, ask and let them know.

On the other hand, there is a response, which is manifested in many ways, such as orgasm and satisfaction. So, it is YOUR partner who will tell you about his/her response. The best responses are sexual pleasure and satisfaction, regardless of orgasm and ejaculation. If you or your partner are not responding, looking for the proper stimuli will help a lot! But, again, the most important thing is what your partner tells you. If your partner says: "I'm happy and satisfy," that will be a good response and enough for you.

Furthermore, between the stimulus and the response, there is a space where you think, perceive, recognize, differentiate, and interpret the stimulus that is coming. Neuroscientist and bestselling author, Dr. David Eagleman suggests that the space between the input (stimulus) and the output (response) is a space for creativity and thinking of possibilities. So, creativity also plays a role in perceiving to respond then. Part of the definition of creativity is that of generating ideas, alternatives, or possibilities, in his case, to respond sexually. Therefore, it is also your responsibility to respond satisfactorily, not just the stimulus provided.

It is something like this:

STIMULUS---*sexual mindset + interpretation + creativity + possibilities*---RESPONSE

Tell your partner what you need and use your creativity, and your sexual mindset to think about various possibilities that will allow you to enjoy and respond with satisfaction!

The Sexual Response Cycle

The sexual response cycle is like an "up and down or back and forth" you and your partner experience when you initiate sexual acts or "go playing." Knowing about the response cycle will help you comprehend the mechanics of sex, so you can relax, enjoy, and enhance the experience and decrease anxiety.

Kim Cattrall and Mark Levinson, authors of *Satisfaction: The Art of the Female Orgasm*, suggest that "starting with gentleness is always best." So, SLOW DOWN when you are about to initiate or "get into" the sexual response cycle. Let's have a brief review of the different models of the sexual response cycle, so you know what you're looking for.

William Masters and Virginia Johnson, during the 60s, were the first to use the term sexual response cycle. They said that the sexual response cycle describes what happens to the bodies of men and women when they become sexually aroused. According to Masters and Johnson, "it refers to the sequence of physical and emotional changes that occur as a person becomes sexually aroused and participates in sexually stimulating activities."

Although there is not only one model of sexual response, the Masters & Johnson model is still commonly used, especially to describe men's response: excitement, plateau, orgasm, and resolution. This is a linear model that "goes up and down," one after the other. See what a linear model might look like:

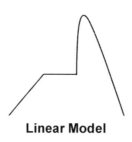

Linear Model

Dr. Helen Kaplan—mentioned in Chapter 2—took this a bit farther in her work in the late 1970s by adding another element as its own phase: Desire. For Kaplan, only 3 phases compose the sexual response cycle: desire, excitement, and orgasm. From there, desire became an essential piece in the sexual response cycle—too important, I would say.

Desire is about the libido, the "I want" piece. According to Kaplan, desire is a mental stage preceding excitement—although not necessarily, according to later models. Kaplan's triphasic model was still a linear model—up and down. So, we can say that we have so far five stages: desire, excitement, plateau, orgasm, and resolution.

In my opinion, nowadays, people pay too much attention to sexual desire or the need for "wanting sex" as being fundamental for sexual activities, forgetting their free will to be sexually connected, regardless of their biological conditions. Women, especially, still emphasize the need for sexual desire as an INDISPENSABLE step or a previous requirement to initiate closeness to their partners. The need for orgasm was another factor for the "successful accomplishment" of these linear models—another more pressure.

In the 90s, Dr. Beverly Whipple—who I had the privilege of meeting, and having a conversation for the first time at a conference in Caracas in 2005—and Dr. Karen Brash-McGreer created and developed a totally new model, a circular model of women's sexual responses. So, the idea of a circular model started to arise. Whipple and Brash-McGreer included more elements in the equation of the sexual response cycle. They included: seduction, sensations, surrender, and reflection, in addition to the existing ones, but now in a circular, continuous way. A circular model is like going "back and forth," never ending. See what a circular model might look like:

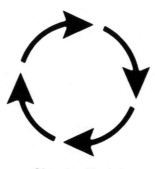

Circular Model

Whipple and Brash-McGreer suggested that "pleasant and satisfying sexual experiences may have a reinforcing effect, leading to the seduction phase of the next sexual experience. If, during reflection, the sexual experience did not provide pleasure and satisfaction, there may not be a desire to repeat the experience." Dr. Whipple stated that women do not necessarily move from one phase of the cycle to the next in a linear way. For example, women can experience orgasm without previous desire, or they can experience desire without orgasm.

Later in the 2000s, Dr. Rosemary Basson reviewed the existence models and added two more elements: emotional intimacy and relationship satisfaction, in the equation of the sexual response cycle. Not only did she add two extremely important elements of human sexuality—emotional intimacy and satisfaction—but she also proposed a non-linear model as Whipple and Brash-McGreer did.

For the first time, a woman's need for emotional intimacy was acknowledged. Circular models are mostly used nowadays, especially to better describe the sexual response of women. Basson believes that people, especially women, have many reasons for engaging in sexual activity other than desire. She acknowledged that desire can be responsive or spontaneous and may come either before or after arousal—in a circular way.

Moreover, Basson also acknowledged that an orgasm is a contributing factor to satisfaction, but not necessary, and she also considered relationship satisfaction. Then satisfaction became the focus point.

Sexual Satisfaction

Neuro-psychotherapist Linda Ohl said that "sexual satisfaction is a subjective term and is solely determined by each individual. For many, feelings of closeness, bonding, touching, and intimacy are enough." The relational aspect of women's sexuality is also now being considered thanks to these circular models. But what happened to the desire phase? It is still an important aspect but it not the sole determiner for connectivity or initiation. As Basson suggested, desire can come after, during, or before sexual activity. So, don't worry about it! The desire for more will follow…as the pressure decreases!

Listening to people, especially women, I hear and see how desire plays a central role in their love lives. I often hear: "I don't have desire, so we don't have intimacy," "I don't feel a sex drive, so we don't have sex," "my partner has more drive than me, I don't have one, so he is angry at me," "she never initiates," "she has not desire at all," and so on. This so-called "a lack of desire" is the result of being stagnant and clung to past outdated ideas and paradigms. Everything we hear around us is shaping our current love lives without us even realizing it.

Kinsey, mentioned earlier, said, "few males achieve any real freedom in their sexual relations even with their wives. Few males realize how badly inhibited they are on these matters." In my opinion, one of the main factors contributing to this fact, still relevant today, is the complicated expectation of sexual desire. How sad it is for people to depend on "the desire for sex"—to be horny—to make love. So, Basson's concept of the circular sexual response fascinates me and reinforces the possibilities of *making love 365 times a year.* Notice that in Basson's model, there are many elements in the equation, but not resolution. There isn't an ending point as in the linear models. It is about engaging anytime in the circuitry of pleasure and keeping yourself there, as long as you want.

And that is precisely the challenge, staying within the cycle, making love. How? Maintaining positive feelings through effective communication, and by using "your stairway." Staying inside the circular cycle of sexual response may be translated into *making love 365 times a year*! You will keep yourselves connected, and your connection will keep you making love.

As the field of sexology has grown, many researchers have added more elements to the equation of sexual response for better understanding of human sexual functioning. One of them is JoAnn Loulan, who smartly added "willingness." In fact, Loulan's model starts with willingness! And that's precisely what you need—the willingness to enter with your partner, holding hands, into the infinite circle of lovemaking. It is time to let go your fears and just enjoy your partner anytime you want because "you do not have to feel desire or be excited to have sex. You only have to have the willingness to have sex," as Loulan says.

More Playing

Another contemporaneous sexologist is Ian Kerner, PhD, mentioned in Chapter 4. He has proposed a model to describe the sex process, which he calls "the Play Process." Kerner mentions three stages in the play process. He has called these three stages: the "Foreplay," the "Coreplay," and the "Moreplay."

We all know what is meant by foreplay and its importance—the warm-up stage. The "Coreplay" is the actual "playing," where you and your partner enjoy sexual activities. Kerner says that Coreplay "doesn't exclude intercourse. But rather is pro-outercourse—a conception of sex that goes beyond penetration embraces mutual pleasure and is better suited to stimulating the female sexual anatomy to orgasm." All kinds of sexual behaviors are "real sex." Then, the "Moreplay"—post-coital time—which many times is missing and means the end of sexual activities for many people. The Moreplay, according to Kerner, is just a break to then continue with more sexual activities, it is not the end of them, since the "play" can continue later…

I love this concept, which coincides with my ideas and suggestions to *make love 365 times a year.* Of course, we all need to rest, take a break, work, be alone, and do things individually and together, etc., but that does not mean disconnection. Staying connected means "keeping the ember active," not necessarily with flames but with enough heat to restart them again, smoothly, easy, and continuously…

Then, you re-start again the playing but with the heat of before and "skillfully extending these foreplay activities into complete, fully realized acts of lovemaking," as Kerner suggests. It is the "game" of transitioning from embers to flames to reach the fire, and to embers again…by always keeping the heat… Remember, you should never leave the "game of love" —your connection to *make love 365 times a year.*

According to studies, more than 60% of couples ignore this magic momentum—the post-coital time or the Moreplay—of being together "keeping the heat" after the playing. Many couples in long-term relationships are missing this momentum. Usually, men just ejaculate, wash up, and go to sleep or leave— and some women too. So bad and sad, because after the "sexual playing" comes the time for snuggling and deepening the connection! The pleasure continues, and so does lovemaking…

A woman in her 30s once told me: "Society has taught us that our sexual satisfaction is not as important as that of man. We have sacrificed our sexual happiness for the well-being of the family, or not to create a scandal, but this has only caused stress, depression, and dissatisfaction. If my husband paid attention to my sexual needs, this could improve my mental health."

As Aliyah from our cases told me after many sessions, "the most important piece of sex for me is not the orgasm, it is the satisfaction I feel now." Orgasm may or may not fulfill you because a woman needs to be emotionally satisfied for pure satisfaction. To rest doesn't mean to stop. You can still touch your partner. The point is the remain connected. As you explore and try new things together, you will learn what your partner likes and what you like and how your sexual response cycle works.

As Basson said: "The best part is the afterglow when we're both limp and glowing with satisfaction, wrapped around each other…the feeling of being so full of him and so full of pleasure that I could explode. The climax of orgasm, whether it's an intense eruption of physical pleasure or an overwhelming emotional sense of being so completely in love with him, brings tears to my eyes."

Together, make sure to commit to "Moreplay" to *make love 365 times a year…*

Part III: Getting Wet

Wetness is an interesting concept in our sex lives; in fact, it has been given the power to measure and even judge whether sexual activities have been good or not, or if a person is fully aroused, full of desire or not, or even if lovemaking was successful! Being wet has been labelled and interpreted as the "sign of sexual desire and arousal," a sign that supposed to means "I want you," or "I am ready,"—you name it…

The truth is natural lubrication is not that important. You should not worry or rate the quality of the sexual response using this variable: being wet. Among women, there is only a 10% of congruence between the sexual experience and the sexual response. That is, natural lubrication may or may not occur regardless of the present sexual experience. So, not lubricating doesn't mean not being sexually aroused and vice versa. Natural lubrication is not an indicator of satisfaction, it is a mechanism that keeps the vagina clean, and protected, that's it.

However, being lubricated or wet is still important to experience sexual pleasure and satisfaction—regardless of if natural lubrication or not. Lubricants are there for you! There is a wide variety of great lubricants, which I recommend having on hand. Remember that the *willingness* to make love is the most essential element. If you aren't wet, don't give up, just get some good lubricant and that's it!

But how wet is wet? The answer is whatever you need. Take your lubricant and use the amount of want so that your experience is very pleasant. Natural lubrication "is by no means an unequivocal indicator that a woman's been amply stimulated. She may be lubricated, but not necessarily aroused…highly aroused, yet not necessarily well lubricated," as Kerner clarifies.

Kissing

What is wetter than a mouth and a deep kiss? Before anything else, a deep kiss should come first! It can't be missed if you want to *make love 365 times a year*! Kissing is a POWERFUL act that brings desire, connection, and pleasure; it's one of my favorite activities and the most erotic way to express passion. Kissing should always be involved in lovemaking! Most people I know and interviewed love deep kissing, especially Hispanics and Mediterranean people. Studies suggest that happy couples French kiss daily, with Italians (75%) kissing the most and having the highest sexual frequency, followed by Hispanics of all ages (72%).

There is a whole science behind the art of kissing. That science or art is called "Philematology." Philematologists have found kissing to be a natural and instinctual mechanism for connection and information. Charles Darwin stated that kissing was natural, an innate part of foreplay. This powerful tool is universal, so much so that studies have found that 90% of cultures around the world practice romantic kissing; only a few don't kiss. Around 46% of the population see kissing as romantic.

The lips hold thousands of nerve endings. It is not a coincidence that the tongue it is used in the two most powerful stimuli: kissing and oral sex—wet activities. The tongue is an important element in sensuality and sexuality, so much so that the tongue is considered an erogenous zone. It's as important as a vulva or a penis. This is the strongest muscle—and unlike your vulva or penis, you can control it and move it as you wish, as slow or as fast, and as wet or dry as you want. You can go over your partner's entire body with it and make them hallucinate! It is a unique wet-phallic organ that never gets old, dry, or tired...

Saliva is there to make your tongue wet and give pleasure and some lubrication. This is important for wet kissing and great oral sex. Kissing is a saliva exchange; saliva has testosterone, a hormone for sexual arousal in both genders. So, you aren't just exchanging saliva; you are exchanging each other's information and hormones!

Fisher—from Chapter 3—says, "kissing evolved to fulfill three essential needs: sex drive, romantic love, and attachment," so kissing plays a role in the each of the three phases mentioned before:

1. Kisses make us desire sex and boost dopamine.

2. Kisses promote romantic love, infatuation and falling in love— and in lust—and boost serotonin.
3. Kissing helps us sustain and strengthen love bonds and keep the connection, and boosts oxytocin, the so-called love hormone.

What about the lips? When the lips and tongues are intertwined, our neural networks are activated. A signal transmits all the nerves of the mouth, lips, and nose to the brain in an instant. We can locate one another's lips in a very dark room, thanks to the brain.

One of the things about kissing is that, you are learning about the quality of your partner. Just by kissing, you may know how compatible your chemistry is. I always say that choosing a partner is 50% chemistry—not what you think about them, but how you feel around them. And, the best way to feel and discover your chemistry is through kissing. You might have to kiss a lot of frogs to find your prince or princess! But how will you know what is good if you don't know what is bad? Learn not through sex, but through kissing—when there are no strange viruses around... Don't have sex just to explore if a person is good for you, because just by dancing and kissing you may find out...that is my suggestion.

The other 50% is compatibility: similarities in relevant areas in life. But wait! Great compatibility and chemistry are not enough, nor do they guarantee that a relationship is going to last and be passionate, healthy, and fulfilling. Work and daily effort are needed, as well. The *7 Sex Secrets* contained in these seven chapters are an attempt to help you sustain a healthy and passionate love life, so you both remain deeply connected.

Good kissing will lead to passion, which is necessary to keep the flames lit. Kissing is the best way to determine how much passion you feel. When you are kissing, you also smelling one another. Remember how important smell is, as discussed in Chapter 6. When kissing, you are combining two senses—smell and taste—to enjoy and learn about one another. In fact, most people close their eyes when kissing, because you do not need your brain to think and tell you what to do, just your senses!

Evolutionary psychologist and researcher from the University of Albany, Robert Gallup, reported that for women the smell and taste of their kissing partner, not the kiss per se, weighed heavily in their decision to continue kissing and pursue a relationship. For them, an unsuccessful first kiss could eliminate a potential partner. Gallup's study also suggested that kissing is more significant for women than for men, is important in both short and long-term relationships, and that men prefer "tongue kissing" over closed-mouth pecks. Overall, women are much more into kissing than men, before, during, and after lovemaking.

Does the role of testosterone in male saliva have something to do with this fact? I think so. This could be a reason why men do not require as much kissing to have sex, as women do. Kissing is not common among female sex workers—men don't need it to get aroused, but women usually do! Women are much less willing to have sex without kissing first. So, if you have a female partner, French kiss her a lot to give her a good dose of testosterone for her libido!

Kissing awakens sexual desire; while not the same as direct stimulation, good kissing may arouse the genital area. If you go to make love without kissing, then you are heading in the wrong direction, on the path to poor sex. Kissing promotes closeness, arousal, passion, and even sexual fantasies. Personality psychologist Jeremy Nicholson, PhD, say, "kissing is a key to love. Kissing can make a partner feel noticed, loved, and connected. This is especially true in long-term relationships, in which kissing can often be forgotten."

So, remember to practice the four kisses habit—once in the morning, once before leaving for work, once when you get back, and once when you go to bed—and Pretzel Time every morning, where you kiss and hug each other before getting out of bed—don't worry about bad breath if you have good dental hygiene. Just kiss! So, kiss your partner every day, "kisses can be ephemeral, or they can leave indelible marks and make you feel more than ever worth living. And although you do not believe it, a kiss, a simple kiss, can change your destiny. It is a key instrument in the symphony of eroticism and life," as Peralta says. Now you know that kissing is an essential element for pleasure and, according to Gallup, "in long-term relationships, the frequency of kissing is a good barometer of the health and well-being of that particular bond." Go ahead and kiss your partner to *make love 365 times a year...*

Now, let's get ready for more wetness... But before we continue, take special note that oral sex, like any other form of sexual expressions, is an act—a sexual behavior or activity—not a person. Sexual activities do NOT determine sexual orientations: heterosexual, homosexual, or bisexual. Sexual orientation is determined by whom you are sexually interacting. The sexual act is what matters now and the technique, not the gender of the people involved—whether receiving or giving.

Oral Sex

You have kissed your partner up; now you need to kiss down! Oral sex is the second most important activity for amazing playing in the bedroom. There is nothing like a wet lick on your genitals. Recall that your wet tongue is an important element for sexual expression, a strong muscle you can control and move as you wish, to make your partner hallucinate! It is a unique wet-phallic organ at your disposal...and saliva is there to bring more pleasure and lubrication...so use it!

When thinking about oral sex, we cannot forget the strength the tongue has and its wonderful virtues to awaken our desires and fantasies and take us to a sensual world of exploration. "There is nothing that compares to the warmth of your breath—the wet sucking of your mouth—the firmness of your tongue," as Sonia Borg, PhD, sexologist and author of *Oral Sex He'll Never Forget*, describes the pleasure of oral activities.

There is a lot of research on oral sex, and I am here not to tell you exactly how to do it, but how important it is for your sex life. The first thing you need to comprehend is that oral sex is real sex, normal, very popular, highly pleasant, and even healthy. But only if you know what you're doing, whom you're doing it to, and why you're doing it. Some of the right reasons to be performing oral sex are:

- ▶ You're with a partner you've chosen, and both of you have agreed and consent to engage in oral sex safely.
- ▶ For pleasure. You both want it and like it or want to learn. You are pleased to please.
- ▶ To arouse your partner during the playing at any time, for fun and more excitement.
- ▶ To orgasm and make your partner sexually happy and satisfied.
- ▶ Because you love each other; lovemaking is about loving each other's entire body, beyond orgasm. As Borg says, "nothing says I love you quite like a blow job... nothing!" It's the same with cunnilingus...

Oral sex has the same name and meaning, regardless of who is doing it to whom. If it is done to a female it is called cunnilingus; if it is done to a male it is called fellatio. The techniques vary, but the rules are the same and apply to any partner, male or female, who is performing the art of oral sex. Likewise, the more you practice, the better you'll be and the more you'll enjoy it—just like with anything else in life! Practice is the key to becoming an expert on anything.

Cunnilingus

First, let's discuss cunnilingus, the art or practice of orally stimulating the female genitals—the vulva. Cunnilingus has the following definitions: "a sexual activity in which female genitals are stimulated by the partner's lips and tongue," "one who licks a vulva, referring to the action, not the actor," and "the oral stimulation of the clit or vulva." The term itself comes from the Latin, "cunnius"—the vulva—and "lingus"—to lick. That is what you are doing—licking a vulva.

Cunnilingus is usually the best and most effective way to get almost any woman to orgasm. Recall that around 80% of women experience orgasm only through clitoral stimulation, and nothing is more direct, precise, and wet than a tongue… So, if you have a female partner, please keep that in mind and eat her vulva! Cunnilingus must be part of the main dish, not just an appetizer…

If you are a woman, or you are with one, learn that other sexual activities like penetration may be very enjoyable, but are probably difficult paths to orgasm, particularly if the clitoris has not been stimulated. Cunnilingus is actual sex and is not inferior to intercourse; on the contrary, in many cases, it is "the only way—beside masturbation—to make a woman experience orgasm," as suggested by Kerner. Take cunnilingus seriously. Learn how to make her come by using your tongue and take all the time she needs for that. Tell your partner how you like it—one of the reasons why masturbation is crucial is that you need to know yourself first in order to teach your partner.

Havelock Ellis, an English physician and expert on human sexuality who wrote the first medical textbook in English on homosexuality, gave his thoughts on cunnilingus, which I consider a tremendous input for us. He said that cunnilingus "tends to be especially prevalent at all periods of high civilization." In my 20+ years of experience, I have observed that educated people have a more open mind about oral sex and enjoy it more. Unexperienced people are a move likely to do it out of obligation and describe the act as nasty or ugly—taboos and restrictions blur the mind.

Fellatio

Fellatio reminds me of gelato, ice cream in Italian. It is orally pleasuring the penis, the phallus. It is the same thing as cunnilingus—oral sex—but on men. The definitions are similar: "oral stimulation of the penis, especially to orgasm," "sexual activity in which the partner's mouth stimulates the penis." Fellatio comes from the Latin "fel," which means to suck and "fellare," "fellatus." References to fellatio can be found in all times and all cultures, from Asian to Greek, and from ancient times to today. Fellatio is commonly known as a blow job.

Unlike for women, oral sex—fellatio—is not, for most males, the main dish; is an appetizer. Don't get me wrong! It is a delightful activity for most of them, they love it, "a blow job in one of the greatest gifts you can give a man," as Borg says, but usually, men don't consider it as the top activity—the most effective way to orgasm—as is intercourse, they are penetrators by nature. In fact, in the huge survey Sex in America, it was found that men reach orgasm during intercourse far more consistently than do women.

However, sometimes blow jobs can be mindblowers, even superior to conventional intercourse. When a blow job is well done (to deepthroating and making him come in your mouth, so you swallow his semen—which is healthy, as discussed in Chapter 2) it can be as delightful as intercourse, or more! Some people don't like to give blow jobs just because they don't know how to do it; not the act per se, but how to get over the feeling of awkwardness. So, your technique is important to do it well, so you're not just doing it, but doing it with passion and the willingness to give pleasure.

So, how do you do it well?!

To help you master either cunnilingus or fellatio, there is a lot of good, updated, and valuable information out there to guide you, like *She Comes First* by Ian Kerner, on cunnilingus, and *Oral Sex He'll Never Forget* by Sonia Borg, on fellatio. These are some of my favorite recommended sources, filled with techniques and suggestions on the art of oral sex. Techniques differ as they are applied to a male or a female. For instance, to hold a penis is easier than to hold a clitoris; or you can't deepthroat a vulva, but you can deepthroat a penis. But in terms of oral sex, certain steps should be followed, for either cunnilingus or fellatio.

Please ALWAYS keep in mind if you are engaging in oral sex—whether cunnilingus or fellatio—during causal sex, or with someone who is not a committed partner, use condoms! Even if it is just oral sex, STDs still can be transmitted this way. Remember, FLUIDS transmit STDs. Stay away from fluids that are not from a committed STD-free partner.

Tips for Oral Sex—Cunnilingus and Fellatio

1. Patience. Especially when performing cunnilingus, women need some time to relax and warm up first—at least 15 minutes. Continue with what you are doing, in a relaxed way; there's no hurry, just take your time to observe changes in your partner's genitals as you lick and suck them. Most women need 20 to 40 minutes of continued, rhythmic, and persistent stimulation to their vulvas—she will tell you where to press—to experience orgasm. During fellatio, the man's penis will get harder and harder. Go SLOW, in both cases! FEEL don't think! Anxiety only brings frustration...

2. Pressure. What is the right amount of pressure? For the clitoris, start very slow and gentle, keeping in constant communication; it will be different for each woman. For him, the penis, keep hold of the base to help determine the right amount of pressure. Apply pressure to his penis with your mouth, lips, and tongue, and avoid involving your teeth.

3. Rhythm. Find the rhythm that works best for your partner and then stick to it. If your partner is responding positively, do not try to change the pace of your licking or sucking, unless they ask you to.

4. Keep it consistent. Trying many different moves is good in the beginning to determine what your partner likes, but when they are close to orgasm, changing tactics will only disrupt this. Breathe and focus only on the rhythm you are in.

5. Enjoy! Don't give up! Keep going; you will get your partner there if you continue your moves as a dance, making sure you express your joy—sexual expressions are hot. Enjoyment and relaxation will help you not to tire, in addition to the expertise that comes with practice. If she orgasms first, it may make intercourse better and may take the pressure off to fully enjoy it.

In fact, she—if you're practicing cunnilingus—will be more open to more orgasms if she orgasms first, so more likely to experience multiple orgasms. Together, you can find the right techniques that work best for you. Every woman and every man are different and have different needs and fantasies. Even when engaging in casual sex, you need open communication, agreement, and an array of techniques to know what will work best. This way, you can become a great lover for your partner.

Manual Sex

Better known as mutual masturbation, manual sex doesn't involve your mouth or your genitals—just your hands. Manual sex is actual sex, too. It is a dry activity where each other's fluids are not part of the playing. This should be a very open activity, with lots of the discussion, as covered previously. Tell your partner exactly how you like to be touched. This is the safest sex of all, as there is no risk for unwanted pregnancy or STDs since there is no fluid contact.

So, I recommend manual sex, especially if you are young and exploring your sexuality. Also, if you have no experience, it is better to start by manually exploring before going far into more sexual acts. Use lubrication and enjoy! Manual sex should be part of your sexual repertoire when making love—a "small sandwich" also counts...because it is still sex.

Penetrative Sex—Penis-in-Vagina Intercourse

It is my opinion that penis-in-vagina intercourse is one of the easiest and most exciting ways to feel each other every day! When you train your body to respond to sensual touches automatically, you are conditioning yourself positively. You can do that through using your senses—smelling, tasting, touching, hearing, seeing—to be ready for lovemaking. Then, when you're close enough, you will be triggering desire just by smelling and kissing your partner—you go LOVEX to make love in an instant. You're already in the Moreplay phase—waiting and wanting... So simple, so beautiful, so exciting! After a while, you'll find yourself *making love 365 times a year* without even realizing it!

Every couple can *make love 365 times a year* in their ways, and you and your partner can do the same, you only need to explore what works for you, as Pedro and I have found. You are learning or reviewing some valid ways of "playing in the bedroom"—3rd Floor—from manual sex to intercourse to find your methods, but always with LOVEX (love, lust, intimacy, passion, and sex—any sexual act).

I always say to my clients; lovemaking should be like food; you always eat, sometimes a little sandwich, other times a big meal, and even a Thanksgiving dinner, but you still eat! With 24 hours in a day, you can take at least half an hour to "eat something" —make love—at any time. Having no time is NOT an excuse! And remember, lovemaking is not about orgasms; it's about connection and pleasure—orgasm is a good bonus.

Sex Positions

Let's explore some positions, because positions are important! Changing positions, especially during intercourse, gives you more time to enjoy and helps prolong the playing, keeping a male partner from ejaculating too quickly. This gives him time to rest and calm down a bit between positions, helping him last longer! The idea is to enjoy and each other.

What about the famous 69 Yes, it is exciting and highly pleasurable, but it is not the best way to experience orgasm. Don't try to have simultaneous orgasms because it only may bring anxiety and frustration. It is only a myth that great lovers have orgasms at the same time. Maybe you will see this in porn, but porn is just adult entertainment, and it is the opposite of what you should do.

Different positions feel different for everyone, and which position you use depends on your needs and many other factors such as body structure, body type, flexibility, healthy issues, weight, and penis-vagina compatibility—including penis size. Other factors, like the surface on which you choose to do it—a bed, a table, a chair, a couch, etc., —may influence position preference as well. Be comfortable; you are not in a porn movie! Be realistic...

The first third of the vagina is where most nerve endings are and where the G-spot is. A woman can experience plenty of pleasure from a 5-inch penis. If your penis or your partner's penis is bigger than 8 inches, be careful when entering; it should be up to her how fast and deep the penis goes. A couple must find what works best for them. Agree beforehand on what you want to do and experience. With any new partner or new position, start carefully and with consent. Go little by little, use lubrication, relax, and enjoy it, and do not suddenly try something different without communicating first.

As we've discussed, oral sex is the best way to provide women orgasms before intercourse. After she has orgasmed, one of the most fabulous ways to initiate intercourse is to penetrate right after her orgasm. Many women love it! In this way, you can create a bridge from experiencing orgasm through clitoral stimulation to experiencing it during intercourse, and have even more pleasure because "man's entry is likely to be far more intense after a long period of great oral sex than without it," suggests by Cattrall and Levinson—mentioned earlier. Try and explore if this works for you. Vigorous intercourse is possible at this point as well as any pleasant sexual activities you prefer; you are in the intense red zone experiencing sexual pleasure. Wait for more and enjoy expressions and moans of passion…

The same is true for same-sex partners, and any type of couples. We are all humans finding and exploring what makes us sexually happy. Sexual pleasure and satisfaction are very individual; the important thing is to find what works for both of you.

There are lots of great books on sex positions, and I am here not to tell you what positions you should adopt, but how important they are for your sex life. *Satisfaction: The Art of the Female Orgasm* by Kim Cattrall and Mark Levinson is a wonderful source to learn more about sexual positions for effective intercourse. However, as Cattrall and Levinson say, "sexual technique is like musical technique. The lover who thinks primarily about technique never really makes love."

Missionary Position

The most famous, common, and conservative of all position: the missionary position. In this position, man is on top, facing the woman, with his penis inside. Although it is the most used, it is the least effective to orgasm. According to Kinsey, for 70% of couples practice this is as the only position they practice. Women are less likely to orgasm this way, especially if the man is rushing. There are variations to this position, like flexing her legs as he leans away from her— possibly even sitting up. This gives a deeper, more pleasurable penetration for her. She will need to move her legs for this; how much, is unique for each couple.

Woman on Top

The most recommended position is woman on top. It is recommended to improve concerns such as rapid ejaculation among other concerns. This will help him control his ejaculation with very little work by grabbing the base of the penis. She also is more likely to orgasm in this position. She can reach her clitoris, and play with, and control the depth of the penis. It is also easier for communication and eroticism because you are face-to-face and can observe each other's expressions of pleasure. This position works well for almost all couples. There are variations to this position as well. Use your imagination and play in your playground!

Sided Entry

Another position is sided entry, or laying to the side, like when you are sleeping. It's the lazy position, where he enters from behind while you are spooning. She may need to adapt her position with her legs. Your morning Pretzel Time cuddling can frequently lead to this position. It can be also face each other, leaning slightly away from each other. This is a comfortable position when you begin intercourse—a fantastic way to start the day!

Rear Entry

One of the most effective, but less-used positions is the rear entry or doggy style position. He is entering her from behind while she is bent over. This can be very exciting and powerful, especially for him, because it gives him a sense of control. She can be quick to orgasm but be careful! Although it is not very intimate since the faces are not seen, it allows deep penetration with the probability of reaching the G-spot and ideally stimulating it. Be gentle and slow as she guides you. Be careful with a large penis or toy; it can quickly become overwhelming or painful for her. Constant communication is key in this position. As with other positions, there are variations to this one, making it hotter. Use your imagination and for playing more!

Anal Sex

Before reviewing anal sex, I want to highlight once again the importance of differentiating sexual behaviors from sexual orientation. Sexual acts don't define your sexual orientation—gay, straight, or bisexual. Just because a person practices oral sex, that does not make them gay, straight, or bisexual. The same is true for the practice of anal sex. Anal sex is another sexual act, like oral sex or penis-in-vagina intercourse, where a phallic object—a penis, a dildo, a finger, a tongue—enters the anus. Now, just because a person practices anal sex, that does not make them gay, straight, or bisexual.

I highlight this concept because it is one of the biggest mistakes and myths I hear. Many people still believe that the practice of anal sex may make a man gay or that is done only by homosexual male couples—a penis in a male anus. Certainly, some gay couples practice anal sex, but they are not the only ones. A heterosexual man does not become gay just because a woman plays with his anus—with a dildo, a finger, a tongue, or anything else. Remember, it is not what you do, but who is doing it to you, and vice versa.

Anyone can practice anal stimulation regardless of their sexual orientation, age, or gender. Some women love it; some don't. Some people only like to stimulate the anus by light touches around it, others like actual penetration. Men, if they are open and relaxed, may find great pleasure from prostate massage and may even experience orgasm. There are lots of great books on anal pleasure; one of them is *Anal Pleasure & Health* by Jack Morin PhD.

Anal sex, or penetration of the anus instead of the vagina, is more popular than you might think. In January 2018, a study found that anal sex is fast becoming an increasingly popular sexual activity among heterosexual couples. Around 36% of women and 44% of men have engaged in anal sex with an opposite-sex partner. Out of all the sexual activities we've discussed in this chapter, anal sex is the riskiest for everyone. The main function of the anus is to expel waste, even though it is highly pleasurable for some. Morin, in *Anal Pleasure & Health*, has made it clear that "the anus is actually one of the human body's most wondrous creations, elegant, efficient, and richly supplied with pleasure nerves."

Here are some rules if you want to explore anal sex:

1. There are three Cs for anal sex: consent, condoms, and cleanliness—both before and after anal sex.
2. It should be a pleasurable activity that can lead to orgasm if wanted. If you feel any strong pain, you must stop.
3. The anus doesn't lubricate itself. Don't just rely on saliva; use plenty of lubrication.
4. Again, use condoms, even if you're just inserting a finger or tongue. Even if the area is clean of waste, bacteria can still linger. Make sure the anus is cleaned before and after anal sex. Sometimes it is recommended to have an enema before anal sex to flush out the area.
5. NEVER penetrate the anus and then penetrate the vagina or mouth immediately afterwards. If you want to switch back to vaginal or oral sex, change condoms and clean the penis first. Anal bacteria in the mouth or vagina can make the recipient very sick. It is better to do oral play and

intercourse before anal sex if you want to—but avoid starting with anal sex, unless it will be the only activity you will do.

6. Don't have anal sex while either partner is drunk. You need to be aware of what your partner is doing! The area is very sensitive and can tear easily.

7. The receiver must be relaxed. The anal muscles will naturally contract when touched; massage around the anus before putting anything inside. The receiver will need to breathe and relax while their partner slowly inserts a finger or small toy little by little to stretch the area, especially if the receiver is a man.

8. Keep your fingernails short and trimmed. This is also true if you plan on using your fingers in the vagina for manual sex. Remember that the anus area is very sensitive and prone to tearing.

Just because you try something new doesn't mean you have to repeat if you don't like it. The important thing is to keep an open mind, explore, and be willing to enjoy playing together while learning more about each other's sexuality.

Orgasm

This is a very interesting and extensive topic, a complex subject that requires knowledge and sensitivity. But, at the same time, it is simple and fascinating, and that is precisely what I want to show you—the simplicity and practicality of the subject.

Let me start by quoting one of my favorite songs that beautifully describes orgasm: *Orgasmo* by Cuban singer Concha Valdes Miranda. What a marvelous way to say what an orgasm is, as Concha Valdes sings: *"Orgasm, nobody wants to mention you, and yet everyone wants to enjoy you…orgasm, who could hold you for more than a moment to die of pleasure and then be reborn…how to say that it is a pleasure and a torment…"*

Yes, orgasm is a highly potent, delightful, and beautiful function of the body to make us happy and healthy! It is a GIFT our bodies have for all of us. At the same time, as the song says, it is a pleasure and a torment because that indescribable moment of joy is too short, leaving us exhausted, and sometimes, wanting more. For some people, that precious gift is challenging to experience for multiple reasons, and one of them is the considerable taboo and negativity people have created around it; as the song says, "nobody wants to mention you."

All humans can experience orgasm; the human body has thousands of nerve endings to allow you to experience orgasms, plus the power of the mind. Orgasm starts and finishes in the brain. Understanding orgasm and its multiple benefits for your overall health—including your immune system— and for your relationship will help you motivate to experience it more often. The world needs MORE LOVE, and that includes more orgasms, instead of fear and pills to treat depression, anxiety, and the unhealthy symptoms that people are suffering today, especially with this horrible virus around us. Nowadays, couples should redefine their relationships to be healthier and more energetic. Problems are opportunities to do better. There should be more information about the potential benefits of experiencing orgasms—regardless of whether you are in a relationship—for our health and well-being. Lovemaking, connection, and orgasms are healthy for you!

Yes, you can live without having orgasms. Maybe that is why medical doctors never ask you if you have orgasms, but what is the quality of life without them? The quality of your love life? What is the impact on your health of not having orgasms regularly? How do you feel when you experience an orgasm? Wouldn't it be nice to have orgasms regularly as part of your health routine? Why not? And, thanks to masturbation or solo sex, we don't need to depend on someone else to experience orgasms…it's totally up to you!

Let's learn a bit what this precious thing is. Remember Aliyah from our case study, who didn't know if she had ever orgasmed. I get this question more than I should. Too often, a woman, and thus her partner, will not know if she has had an orgasm, especially young or inexperienced women. So, what is an orgasm?

The Science of Orgasm

The word orgasm comes the Latin and Greek word orgasmo meaning "organ to grow ripe." The Webster definition is, "the rapid pleasurable release of neuromuscular tensions at the height of sexual arousal." And, a more scientific definition comes from Drs. Barry Komisaruk, PhD, and Beverly Whipple, PhD, in which they describe orgasm as, "a peak intensity of excitation generated by a) Afferent and re-afferent stimulation from visceral and/or somatic sensory receptors activated exogenously and/or endogenously, and/or b) higher-order cognitive process, followed by a release and resolution (decrease) of excitation. By this definition, orgasm is characteristic of, but not restricted to, the genital system."

Orgasm, then, is the sudden release of tension as a response to a stimulus, strong enough to produce such response, which is expressed by involuntary, fast and rhythmic contractions in the genital area, typically around 5 to 15 contractions in 10-20 seconds, involving the whole body. That is true for both women and men. That's orgasm, available to all!

The tension-building leads to sudden, rough hotness inside and a feeling of great release. If you are cold and sleepy, getting aroused will raise your body temperature and wake you up. And, usually, having an orgasm will shake your entire body, from head to toes, for a very fleeting moment. Men and women—and all people—are different. We are all different, so everyone will experience orgasm in many different intensities and ways and triggered in diverse ways. But the fact is that we all were born with this capacity, and orgasm is orgasm.

Experiencing Orgasm

Women, as well as men, need to RELAX first to be able to perceive, and enjoy the stimulus provided—whether by yourself, with your partner, with or someone or something else. If your body needs an orgasm—a release—you probably will feel desire to orgasm and it will be easier. Also, your body and your mind can even trigger the response by having an unexpected orgasm, as a natural respond of your body, especially while sleeping.

Remember, how previously we talked about the stimulus leading to perception—imagination—creativity to then, response. So, to experience an orgasm, you need a stimulus (what turns you on). Secondly, you need some imagination and positive perception in order to get highly aroused so you can build enough tension to then release it. The response—the sudden involuntary release of the tension built—will be expressed by involuntary fast contractions: orgasm. This process is the same for everyone (men and women) but manifested in diverse ways.

The stimulus—what causes such a response—is NOT the same for everyone and sometimes can bring you lots of trouble. The truth is, as I say, you don't need a relationship to have orgasms; you just need the time to make yourself orgasm through masturbation! A relationship is for a lot more than that, and if you share your orgasms with your partner, then it will be much better!

However, you DO need a partner to make love! Lovemaking is far beyond experiencing orgasms. It is about the deep sharing of energies and a connection that has no scientific definition as an orgasm does, and its benefits transcend our human knowledge... Of course, orgasms are welcome as a result.

Female and Male Orgasm

Studies show that the type of relationship, and its duration, have an impact on female orgasm. Around 67% of women have an orgasm when they are in a stable relationship after six months or more, and only 11% achieve orgasm during the first sexual encounter. When faking an orgasm, a woman may be doing fast contractions or Kegels, but in a true orgasm, the vaginal contractions happen too fast to be faked. Doing Kegel exercises might fool your partner—particularly if they are inexperienced—but you cannot fool yourself. And you will feel them for sure! Wait, relax, and let go!

On the other hand, men may fake orgasm as well, but they usually don't need to since the focus is always on his ejaculation and not his orgasm. In fact, when a man says he has experienced orgasm but hasn't ejaculated, his partner usually won't believe it, because he is a man and men ejaculate. Some people even believe that a man needs to ejaculate—otherwise, he has a problem. Many women even get angry if their male partner doesn't ejaculate in each sexual encounter, even if he's had an orgasm...

Men feel the same as women during their orgasms. In the brain, their responses are the same, and they will likewise feel a few fast and involuntary contractions and the release of tension during orgasm. Now, most men need direct stimulation of the penis—their main sex organ—via manual sex, oral sex, and/or intercourse to experience orgasm. Most women need direct stimulation of the clitoris and/or the areas around it, through oral or manual sex. Some women can experience orgasm by indirect stimulation of the clitoris, vaginal stimulation, or even by thinking. New research has suggested that the clitoris is the epicenter of orgasm, regardless of how and from where it was triggered.

Any way is a valid way to experience an orgasm. There is no better orgasm; orgasm is orgasm, and they all bring lots of pleasure to men and women, regardless of how it was triggered—the type of stimulation rather than the type of orgasm. Whipple has made great contributions by re-discovering the G-spot, named after German researcher Ernst Gräfenberg, who first identified it. It brings intense pleasure and not necessarily orgasm. The best way to explore it is with a finger 2 inches inside the vagina, touching the top. Orgasms can be trigged by proper stimulation of the G-Spot as well.

What about having more than one orgasm simultaneously or multi-orgasms—is it possible? YES! It is possible, especially for women. Both men and women have the potential to experience multi-orgasms. Women can learn and train themselves to experience more than one orgasm at a time. It requires total surrender and letting go! Men can experience more than one orgasm before ejaculating. For men, it is all about self-knowledge and training. This is possible if you know very well your body and have control over your ejaculation.

Understand that orgasm and ejaculation are not the same thing. Men can experience orgasm without ejaculating when they have trained themselves. The opposite is also true. It has been documented that a man can ejaculate without experiencing orgasm, which means that he did not enjoy himself or have pleasure, and therefore, he usually evaluates the experience as unsatisfactory despite having ejaculated.

Some Benefits of Orgasm

Whipple and Komisaruk, and many others have made a huge contribution as well on the impact orgasms have in the brain—yes, not only in your body, but in your brain. They found that during orgasm, lots of brain centers become active, even otherwise unused parts. As I said, orgasms are a blessing and a gift, which can help you heal from depression and many other situations. And, they bring great pleasure, connection, joy, and bliss when making love. Shelley's book, from Chapter 2, is a great source to learn more about the benefits of orgasm—so can be motivated to experience more orgasms. And who enjoys more orgasm? You guess it! Men!

It is perhaps not surprising to learn of Dr. Fredrick's findings, published in the Archive of Sexual Behavior, that men in heterosexual relationships have the greatest number of orgasms. The group with the least number? Women in heterosexual relationships. In fact, women in heterosexual relationships were found to have far fewer orgasms than women in same-sex relationships. It was also found that people receiving oral sex have more orgasms and higher sexual satisfaction than those that don't.

But there is no doubt that men are more ready to have sex and experience orgasm than women. It is not better or worse; it is what it is!

Ejaculation

Some women can ejaculate—the so-called female ejaculation, commonly known as *squirting.* This isn't exactly an orgasm, per se; it can happen before, during, or after orgasm. A gush of liquid that isn't urine comes from the urethra when the G-spot is properly stimulated by fingering, a toy, or a penis. While urine particles might be found in this liquid, it is not urine, it is safe, clean and should be enjoyed! Squirting is another response that comes from proper stimulation. Plenty of books and videos explain how to stimulate the G-spot.

Although it is still a controversial topic, I think all women should explore it and find out what gives them pleasure. Trust, confidence, relaxation, and surrender are essential to explore beyond your sexual comfort zone. But women don't need to ejaculate; it is just an experience to enjoy if they want to. Female ejaculation seems not to be common among all women, and it is not linked to orgasm. Unlike women, all men—in healthy conditions—ejaculate and should do so with a certain frequency, to keep the system clean. Ejaculation is different than orgasm and has a different process that involves different parts and circuits. Male ejaculation is the expulsion of semen through the urethra, right after the contractions.

It is so close to orgasm that it is very difficult to differentiate two. Men have a very hard time differentiating orgasm from ejaculation. Because of that, plus the lack of positive sex education, most men are not aware of this fact, and some find it too hard to control themselves to be able to separate the two. Some have trained themselves to the point of enjoying great and extended pleasure and lasting as long as they want. Ejaculation for them is under control most of the time, and no longer a problem. They can experience orgasms first, and ejaculate when they want, which doesn't mean they cannot ejaculate—these are two different things.

Don't get me wrong, I know men find absolute great pleasure ejaculating; it is healthy and very pleasurable. I am just saying that the two are different, so you, as a man, need to master your own body and find ways to experience high pleasure and satisfaction as the ultimate goal! Remember, female ejaculation is the exception not the rule, whereas male ejaculation is the rule, not the exception.

Dr. Willian Hartman and Marilyn Fithian, founders of the Center for Marital and Sexual Studies, did extensive research on male orgasm. They found out that "the strongest impediment most men must overcome when they think of multi-orgasms for themselves is the belief that orgasm, and ejaculation are inextricably bound together. Ejaculation and male orgasm are not synonymous. We do not expect male orgasm to be always accompanied by ejaculation. Men could—if they learned how—have as many orgasms as women do during one sexual experience."

Every person is unique and has their own way of responding sexually and expressing their own sexual satisfaction. The common factor is that every woman and man need effective stimulation in order to orgasm. Specific actions, thoughts, and fantasies are unique everyone who experiences orgasm, but the most important element is your intimacy because "success in sex is ultimately determined by intimacy—not by the number of orgasms each partner experiences," as Hartman and Fithian said.

Hartman and Fithian have defined orgasm "as a peak in emotional and physical responses, accompanied by pelvic contractions, experienced during sexual stimulation. Similarities between male and female sexual responses are far greater than most people expect them to be." Learn about your body and help your partner learn what is an effective stimulus for you. Go for a good playing together and *make love 365 times a year*—which doesn't mean you have to have 365 orgasms and/or ejaculations a year—if you want, and can, go ahead, but it's not what I mean.

Lovemaking goes far beyond the technicality of orgasm; it is an expression of love and the most intimate connection. The communion of those who love each other when they join and merge their souls through the contact of their lips and skin. As sex therapist and author Judith Sachs says, "the sexual act is only a small part of your sexuality. People who care about each other tend to value their common interests...and have the ability to experience a range of emotions together."

Part IV: Sexual Enhancements

Now that you have all the elements to stay connected and make love, you can add a delicious cherry on top of your cake. Now that you and your partner have built a solid Three-Floor house, it is time for some enhancements that may spice up your love life, if you want, with different sexual scenarios—different touches and tastes that sweeten and enrich your 3rd Floor. Notice I am saying "the cherry on top," not the cake itself… Without a cake, there is no place to add the cherry, right? So be aware that ANY sexual enhancement is to enrich your love life, not to fix it, substitute it, destroy it, or replace it.

Remember from the beginning of this chapter that, many couples with sex and relationship problems tend to jump straight to the mechanics of sex or enhancements to solve their love conflicts. But they will be very disappointed when trying different things like sex toys, trips, and threesomes—cherries— without a cake. So, improve any existing conflict and find ways to connect to your partner first and be happy together before introducing any extra external help like enhancers. They work wonderfully and are great when you want to boost experiences.

What are enhancers? According to the definition, an enhancement is a change, or a process of change, that improves something or increases its value. That's exactly what we want now—lovemaking with even more lust, and to the best of your ability with more passion!

Enhancers are objects and activities that may make your sexual experiences even more pleasurable and boost your passion. Especially in long term relationships, couples can struggle to keep sex fresh and new. Here are some suggestions to enhance your sex life—things to boost pleasure in your 3rd Floor. These aren't things you would do naturally; you need to be conscious and aware of what you're doing. They should never take the place of meaningful connections; sexual enhancements only enrich the stimulus to boost the response—creativity is your first ally. You'll be focusing on the stimuli itself to better the response through your creativity. I've said it before and will say it again now: for a healthy experience, sex needs to be consensual, safe, responsible, and pleasurable—Chapter 2.

The number one enhancer is lubricants and then, sex toys to boost any sexual experience. So, always include:

1. Lubricants
2. Potent sex toys
3. Condoms (if you aren't in a committed relationship)

Always have lube nearby; this is a must for anal sex and sex toys, and especially if she is past menopause. Even if she is aroused, she may not have enough lubrication. Lubes are great enhancements that should never be missed. They help women—and men—feel more comfortable.

There are two kinds of lubes: silicone-based, and water-based. Silicone-based lasts longer and is good for long periods of intercourse (penis-in-vagina or anal) or if you are having sex underwater, such as in a pool, bathtub, or in the ocean. Water-based is best when using sex toys and some condoms. Lubes are your best friend!

Sex Toys

For about three years, I contributed to Cali Exotics, doing reviews about different sex toys. Cali Exotics is one of the largest and best sex toy stores in America. They used to send me the newest sex toys, and I would review them. I loved them all! I ended up with so many I gave them out as Christmas presents! Sex toys are great, and they are good for women, men, and couples. They can be expensive, so you need to know what you want before shopping, but it is worth it!

I have read many studies and have written many articles about sex toys. There is not a single study against *good-quality* sex toys; on the contrary, all good-quality are positive! Couples that use sex toys rate higher on levels of pleasure and sexual satisfaction. Sex toys are NOT the enemy! They will not replace a penis, a partner, or become addictive. They are helpers only to enhance your sexual response. Sex toys don't have to be there every time in every playing; they should be used for a variety, on special occasions, or to enrich an experience. However, there are cases where the use of sex toys is indispensable, as in the case of people with certain disabilities. We all have the right to enjoy sexual pleasure...

My research found that sex toys boost sexual encounters—the playing—and make any experience more pleasurable in diverse ways. Moreover, researchers have found that women who use sex toys have more orgasms, easier and faster. In fact, sex toys help couples to maximize their orgasmic potential. The only negative thing I have found is how expensive sex toys can be! Other than that, there are no downside. You can find sex toys for women, for men, and for all couples.

Vibrators

The most popular sex toys are vibrators, especially for women. But they can also be used on men. They can stimulate the scrotum and help relax the anus. But mainly vibrators are used on the clitoris. They can help women who have difficulty orgasming because a vibrator has different abilities than a tongue or finger. Start with the vibrator on a low setting before slowly intensifying it. It will awaken the clitoris and can be turned up until she experiences orgasm.

Vibrators can be found in all shapes and sizes, even as small as a tube of lipstick. If you're embarrassed about buying a vibrator, they can be small and discreet and ordered online. The boxes will be brown and unmarked. Small vibrators can be hidden inside panties, and some come with a control for the partner to use. Some are even waterproof! Sex toys are a big industry right now, and updates are always being released.

You can use vibrators to warm up before the playing or intercourse. They are for external use only, not to be inserted into the vagina. The best way of experiencing orgasm when masturbating is with a vibrator. Vibrators can be used during solo sex or with a partner(s). During intercourse, use the toy on her clitoris while he is inside of her—both will experience pleasure!

Dildos

Dildos are sex toys with a penis shape that are to be inserted into the vagina or anus. They can be used on a man or a woman. Both heterosexual and homosexual couples can use dildos, but, in ALL cases, make sure to use lube as well. Like vibrators, dildos come in all shapes and sizes, but most will be shaped like a penis. Small dildos can find the G-spot, they usually aren't as big as a penis and can be easily angled. There are dildos that are also vibrators, where the vibrator is on the side of the dildo.

There are also sex toys that can improve a woman's PC muscle. Most toys have batteries or need to be charged, if they have a vibrating aspect. If you want them to do something specific—like find the G-spot or work the PC muscle—make sure you look for that feature while shopping. Toys for men include toys that can suck or envelop the penis. You can have some fun without using your mouth! There are also small dildos for prostate stimulation, with or without vibration.

When is a great time to use sex toys? Any time! A great occasion can be when women are on their period, put a towel down, and use the toys to have an orgasm. Some women have a higher sex drive during their period and are naturally horny from the hormones. This is a less messy way to bring about orgasms during that time. It's also great if their partner is tired. You can use the toy to help your partner without doing much work. These toys aren't here to destroy anything, but to do amazing things! It is not reasonable to think a sex toy will replace your partner. This is a very old-fashioned mindset. A sex toy will NEVER compete with a partner; it is simply a tool to be used to enhance the experience.

Selecting your vibrator or dildo is a fun activity! You can go to the store or use the Internet. I recommend Cali Exotics, but there are many other great companies to find good-quality sex toys and other fun things to enjoy together. If you feel uncomfortable, using the Internet is always an excellent choice. Get a good quality toy and keep it clean. Wipe it with a wet cloth before and after use.

Talk to your partner and visit sex shops together. Using sex toys is part of your sexual intimacy and is very erotic. Don't be shy; sex toys are normal and healthy. Together, pick the best toy for the two of you. There are a large variety of sex toys for men and women. My recommendation is to get silicone toys; they last longer and are usually higher quality (just remember to use water-based lube with it!).

Beyond Vanilla

Sex toys help or enhance the response. A kinky style enhances the stimulus or is the stimulus. It is sexual playfulness to make your playing diverse and hot. There are sex games you can play with your partner to stimulate your sex appetite. There are card games that can give you some ideas and spice up the moment. Trying something new and different doesn't mean this is now your lifestyle or a unique stimulus you must incorporate. To explore beyond your boundaries just means to have experienced something new, not that you have become such-and-such or have changed your love-style.

There is a difference between experience and lifestyle. Differentiating what an experience and lifestyle are can bring you comfort, and freedom to explore more. Nobody changes their love-style or orientation because they have experiences outside the conventional. Experiences, and going beyond your comfort zone may bring you more knowledge about yourself and your partner, plus more pleasure and an even deeper connection.

Going a little farther if you want, you and your partner can try different activities—including different objects, toys, places, or even other people. It's all about going beyond the conventional methods. Vanilla sex is considered conventional sex. It is, for instance, penis-in-vagina intercourse. It is very hard to cross a line between conventional sex or vanilla, kinky style, or non-vanilla sex.

As always, it is not black or white; there is a huge spectrum of colors, variations, and depth. From foot fetishes, high heels, lingerie, role playing, cross-dressing, and rough intercourse to spanking, BDSM, threesomes, and group sex, there is a large menu to enjoy each time you want it, going out of your conventional vanilla sex to something else…

Am I kinky?

The *7 Sex Secrets* still apply to non-vanilla and open relationships. If you have a committed partner, or primary partner, you should make sure you communicate very well, don't hold resentment, and that both of you are happy and connected. Otherwise, you will have conflicts that will prevent you from enjoying each other and will not respond positively. Remember that a sexual response occurs from a sexual stimulus and its interpretation. If you are upset, distrustful, insecure, or anxious, you will block the response. You require serenity, confidence, security, and trust in yourself and in your partner to be able to enjoy and be "confidants." Effective communication is essential when exploring new ways and novel situations.

If you don't have a committed partner yet, choosing the right partner will bring you serenity. A right partner is not a perfect person with no problems—that doesn't exist. It means someone suitable for you and your love-style. When dating someone you like, avoid lying or hiding your love-style; you will not change anyone over time, you will only bring conflict and pain. The best thing is, to be honest (to yourself first), respectful, and open to share your love-style (vanilla, non-vanilla, open, or closed, or whatever) with confidence and pleasure, and without conflicts. Find someone like you! That is the key to a successful relationship, regardless of styles and orientations.

Boundaries

Set your boundaries! Boundaries—physical and emotional—are healthy and protect us. You and your partner need to know what is wanted, and how, and when, as well as and your specific limits. The more you want to explore, the more communication and boundaries you need to have. As best-selling author Thomas Gagliano says, "we don't practice a fire drill when there is a fire. Similarly, when setting boundaries, the person needs to practice what boundaries they need to set before they implement them. Without healthy boundaries, we hurt each other, and we allow ourselves to be hurt by others."

With that in mind, let's look at some common non-vanilla styles. But before exploring any style, make sure you are both ready and interested! Again, communication is truly key here, as well as the four main rules about healthy sex: consensual, safe, responsible, and pleasurable. Some non-vanilla options to explore are:

▶ Role playing with different sexual scenarios and dressing-up in all different styles. First, agree to do it; don't do this as a surprise at the beginning. Once you establish your role play, you can add variety to your repertoire and surprise your partner. If you wear the same clothing every time, it'll fall apart. Use variation!

▶ Light bondage, including blind-folds, and cuffs, where you tie one another up, taking turns, or blindfold your partner, can be an exciting experience. It requires a lot of trust. Erotic massages with stimulating oils while being blind folded to happy endings.

▶ Quickies in forbidden, strange or unusual places like an airplane, car, train, the beach, at the back yard, while camping, in your neighbor's bathroom, in the theater watching live sex, or in the rain. Quickies are best used when having adventurous sex in weird places. Having quick, controlled sex occasionally is not a problem. This doesn't mean rapid ejaculation. Try to create the sensation of being caught while not actually getting caught. I do hear a lot of people having this kind of adventurous sex with strangers—this is very risky! But if it's with a partner, it is not risky. Be responsible and know what you are doing.

▶ Spanking, scratching and biting as you both like and agree to. Rough sex can be very stimulating for some people.

▶ Dominance and submission (DS). Whether you want to dominate or be dominated, these specific roles can be very stimulating. They are about power exchange. Both partners need to be clear and agree before the playing. Forced sex, is a common sexual fantasy, but it is not real rape— just the thought of being abused by agreement!

▶ The practice of voyeurism (if you like to watch). This does not mean to watch or spy on people without agreement—that's not consensual! You can go to places to watch live sex or strip teases or watch porn and erotic movies together—that's consensual. The same is true for exhibitionism (if you like to be watched), which doesn't mean to annoy others without consent. You can go to places where, by consent and agreement you can get naked or perform a strip tease, or you can film (carefully) yourselves if you both consent it.

▶ BDSM is a variety of erotic practices or roleplaying involving bondage, discipline, dominance and submission, sadomasochism, and other related interpersonal power exchanging dynamics. Some people role playing and use this practice to stimulate themselves. Others consider BDSM as a lifestyle in which they self-identify as belonging to this specific community. So, it ranges from light experiences to a lifestyle. BD refers to bondage and discipline, DS refers to dominance and submission, and SM refers to sadism and masochism. Even the strongest BDSM lifestyle playing is by consent of the people involved. Communication, agreements, and boundaries are fundamental. This is not about abuse— abuse is not consensual. This is a consensual lifestyle, practice, or experience.

Opening Your Relationship

Opening a closed relationship means moving beyond having sex with only your partner to having sex with other people outside your relationship, by agreement. In a recent study published in the Journal of Sex and Marital Therapy, it was found that about 10% of couples in the USA are engaging in some form of open relationship; that is, 10% of couples are having sex with other people.

What is an open relationship? Let's understand first what monogamy is. Monogamy means: One=*mono* and partner=*gamy*—so, one partner. Helen Fisher, from Chapter 3, has stated: "Monogamy is natural. In every single culture in the world, most men and women in every 'household' have one man and one woman. We do not share naturally; we are a monogamous species. We got a brain circuitry for it. We got tremendous brain pathways to fall in love and to attach to a partner. Yes, we are monogamous animals." Yes! It means that we want and need to be paired!

Therefore, we all have the drive to form a pair-bond, to have one partner. In the past, one partner in a lifetime; nowadays, one partner at time, which is referred as serial monogamy. I share the view of clinical psychologist Dr. Alicia Clark that we don't set out to have sexual relationships with other people. The thing is that we forget about our mate (we no longer pay attention) and do very little to keep things fun, alive, and exciting with them. Then we find in other people what we haven't cultivated in our own relationship. See? You just are seeking out adventure, fun, connection, validation, sex, and whatever is missing in your relationship or in your life. But still, you will want to be in a relationship by nature. So, being monogamous is natural!

On the other hand, fidelity is not natural, as Fisher says, "fidelity is a choice." It is the choice we make to respect and keep agreements with our partner. It is a task, a task we need to successfully perform and respect. One definition of fidelity is "strict observance of promises, duties, etc. Honest or lasting support, or loyalty, especially to a partner. Faithfulness to a person, cause, or belief, demonstrated by continuing loyalty and support." I think it is essential to understand that fidelity is not a natural drive; it is a cognitive decision that requires some thinking, evaluation, and decision-making. If you leave it in autopilot, the natural outcome will be the opposite—infidelity, forgetting your agreements.

Many times, monogamy is confused with fidelity—if you are monogamous, then you are faithful—which is not true. This assumption can be very dangerous, leading to lots of problems, and terrible feelings (Chapter 3) because these are two different things. Many couples assume when they become committed that fidelity will occur naturally, that they are going to remain faithful to each other, no matter what, without in putting any effort (you can explore infidelity in Chapter 3).

Therefore, these couples don't talk about their needs and never discuss the possibilities of temptations, attractions, and the need for novelty, uncertainty, and variation. They form a relationship without specific rules and agreements. What a mess! Heterosexual couples in close relationships often fail to do so, taking for granted this type of conversation, making their rules very blurry, unspecific, and implicit.

A close relationship is when a couple agrees on being exclusive to each other sexually and emotionally. An open relationship is when a couple, by agreement, decide not to be sexually and/or emotionally exclusive. So, there are many types of agreements and variations in which couples decide in what ways they are going to be exclusive or non-exclusive. Breaking these rules and agreements makes is what makes you unfaithful, not the fact of being in an open or in a closed relationship; infidelity can occur in an open relationship as well.

Nurturing Your Relationship—Open or Closed.

Sometimes you may have a hard time cultivating your relationship and keeping your focused ATTENTION on your partner. As Fisher says, "we have all the equipment to be in love and attach to one partner"—at a time. But it seems that for some people it is very difficult, either because they don't know how, or they don't want to make efforts, leading to infidelity, lies, betrayal, and the many problems that follow. There are many reasons a person is unfaithful, even in happy relationships, and one of them is the tendency to think about our needs, forgetting our partner.

To be sexually and emotionally exclusive and faithful, you need to provide the best possible environment for each other. Provide some novelty, uncertainty, and excitement; make it fun and hot while still secure and certain, not forgetting your partner at any moment. Cultivating passion is a task as well as keeping the lust, and especially making an effort to pay attention to each other to keep the connection. In other words, you need to have LOVEX—whether if you are in a closed relationship or not.

When a couple in a closed relationship decides to open their relationship, it means they are agreeing on being not exclusive in a certain way. Since there is such a huge diversity and so many variations and ways to open a relationship, it is very important to discuss what you want and expect first with your partner. Communication here is KEY. Sit and TALK first!

Types of Open Relationships

Studies have found that couples in open relationships have a higher degree of trust and better communication than couples in closed relationships. Less surprisingly, they also have more sex—not necessarily lovemaking. There is a wide variety of open styles today: threesome, foursomes, swinging (only sexually open), polyamory (sexually and emotionally open to specific people), group sex, and many other styles, varieties, and degrees of openness.

Sex columnist Dan Savage refers to couples in closed relationships who occasionally, open their relationship—by agreement—to explore and go playing with other people. Savage suggests that these kinds of agreements are becoming popular among straight couples across the country. People aren't talking about it, but it is more common than you think! This means making some room for others, in different times and different ways, in specific occasions, while remaining closed. For some couples, it may only happen while traveling or at certain times of the year, as an enhancer.

Social psychologist Art Aron, PhD, found that exciting, novel, and challenging activities together—as a couple—can make a huge difference in the quality of your love life and relationship. Some couples have found it very exciting the playing with people outside the relationship, occasionally. What if you decide, or have already decided, to open your relationship as a lifestyle? Fine, but you still have a primary partner, and this book can still help you *make love 365 times a year.* Threesome, foursomes, group sex, swingers, and other types of openness can also be a lifestyle, not just an experience.

Swinging is a lifestyle where couples have already fully opened their relationship. The agreements vary, but they are usually emotionally exclusive but sexually non-exclusive. They explore sex with others while expanding their boundaries. Swingers share only according to their agreements.

Polyamory is another lifestyle in which a couple share and choose other couples or individuals to be part of their relationship, to share not only sexually but emotionally as well. A simple definition is that "polyamory is openly, honestly, and consensually loving and being committed to more than one person." They are people in open relationships. The interesting fact is that these couples are beyond sexual and emotional exclusiveness; they share their duties, chores, finances, and social and domestic lives as a big family of 2, 3, 4 or more. It is like being married and committed to multiple people! Well, they are in their own way.

They are consensual, and all participants have agreed. Unless a partner breaks the rules, they are not cheating or lying. Again, open communication and boundaries are fundamental here, and being in an open relationship is a choice.

Think Again

Always, before you decide how to enhance your sexual experiences, you must communicate well, be sure about your relationship, and be well connected to your partner. Exploring without precaution can go from being an exciting experience to a disaster, ending in frustration and break ups—as in many cases—because "being open to different partners it is just not what we can live with well," says family therapist Sara Kay Smullens.

Keep working on your relationship, find the time to have regular exciting dates with your partner, and novelty time as well. If you decide to experience with other people, build first thoughtful conversations, clarification, and careful consideration, to enhance your love life and to learn from each other, not to destroy and ruin your life.

Remember that lovemaking is not about "fucking other people," it is about loving your partner with a naked soul. The soulmates do not exist; they are not "born or found;" you both create an ideal "soulmate" relationship with effort! You become soulmates when you make love... Touch, kiss, Pretzel, your partner, and enjoy *making love 365 times a year*—sometimes with orgasm and sometimes not. Build a beautiful great, fun, and solid Three-Floor House with a fantastic 3rd Floor full of LOVEX!

And keep in mind Fisher's wise suggestion: "If you want a good sex life, HAVE SEX, it is going to trigger those brain systems for romantic love, attachment, and sex drive." Find the best ways to enhance your love life because there's only one life, and you are alive!

> "Sex is emotion in motion."
>
> —Mae West

Part V: 7 Simple Suggestions & Recommended Sources

7 Simple Suggestions for Enhancing Your Love Life

1. Kiss your partner daily; make sure you have at least one French kiss per day, using your tongue, lips, and your whole mouth. Enjoy your partner's saliva; smell and feel them. Your mouth is highly sensitive and erotic; your lips have tons of nerve endings. This is the most powerful way to initiate "the playing" and continue with it. Deep kissing with passion is:

    a. EXPLORATORY: By kissing, you know your partner and transmit information to each other.
    b. BONDING: Oxytocin levels (the attachment hormone) highly increase.
    c. STIMULANTING: You are stimulated sexually and prepared for passionate sex.

d. HEALTHY: Increases the production of saliva. You activate 34 muscles and strengthen your immune system when French kiss!

So, kiss more! Kiss, kiss, kiss! Surprise your partner with an unexpected kiss—this is best in the morning before leaving. Give a short but intense wet, warm kiss. Gently bite the lower lip, enter with your tongue just a little, smell their face, and breath in their ear. Repeat when meeting again at the end of the day, but longer and more intense...

2. If you are *not* in a committed closed relationship —sharing with only one partner, known to be uninfected—USE A CONDOM! Always use a condom when practicing oral, vaginal, or anal sex to avoid transmission of STDs. Stay away from FLUIDS if you are not sure or do not have a condom; just practice manual sex. Be careful with cuts and fluids. Be clean and enjoy yourself wisely.

3. Explore each other's bodies and genitals. Start by touching each other's faces, gently and slowly, to feel and connect. Explore each other's bodies using your fingers and say tender words to each other. Intercourse is not the only way to penetrate; meaningful words deeply penetrate each other's souls. So, intercourse does not only occur with a penis; it also occurs with tender words and tender hearts.

4. An active and satisfactory sex life is about the subtle combination of sexual tension, relaxation, enjoyment, and satisfaction. Think about sex during the day and initiate small plays at every opportunity, not only right before having sex or in the bedroom. Touch your partner in an erotic manner when you are out together, like in the car, in a bar, or restaurant, while walking, or in activities together, so you warm up and accumulate some sexual tension for later. Don't wait to be in bed; start and continue your foreplay throughout the day. Then, don't avoid sex. Have sex, initiate foreplay, and *make love* at least once a day.

5. Practice oral sex frequently to get better and better master it! Be patient and SLOW DOWN. Taking your time and finding a comfortable position is key to oral sex, for truly enjoying and pleasing your partner. Be sure you are clean. Hygiene is crucial. Remember that cunnilingus

is an excellent way to make a woman come, to enjoy her vulva. Fellatio is also highly desirable. Try at least once to the deep throat his penis and make him come in your mouth. Swallow all his cum. Not only it is good, it is healthy. Remember all the many benefits of semen. Semen is pure and very healthy when a man eats healthy and does not smoke. Semen is a protein fluid rich in potassium, iron, calcium, lecithin, vitamin E, phosphorus, many proteins, and testosterone and other hormones and essentials. It is anti-anxiety, anti-cancer, and anti-depressant.

6. A wide repertoire of SEXUAL POSITIONS is a key element in the art of making love. Many couples say they only use between two and three positions; the typical three: 1. Man on top (the Missionary), 2. Woman on top (Superior), and 3. Side to side (Perfumed Garden-Kama Sutra). The woman on top position is great for both partners, giving her greater stimulation and free access to the clitoris while he enjoys watching her. These are not the only positions; everything depends on your CREATIVITY, CONFIDENCE, and the PHYSICAL CONDITIONS of the participants. The important thing is to experiment and vary your activities in bed, which keeps the passion alive and drives away boredom. Include more than three positions in your routine. Novelty brings connection!

7. Your sexual energy is limitless and, renewable, and is enhanced with sexual activity. The more active you are, the more likely you are to be sexually active and enjoy sex years later, in old age. Sexual activity is not an extra activity in your life that exists only for procreation, to please your partner, or for special occasions "to celebrate." Lovemaking should be an important, vital, and essential part of your daily life. It will bring you wellness to help you live your healthiest, most vibrant life, with joy and pleasure, as well as to rejuvenate, beautify and strengthen yourself and your love life. *Make love 365 times a year* and connect!

Recommended Sources for Sex Secret #7

Kissing by Andrea Demirjian

The Science of Orgasm by Barry R. Komisaruk, Carlos Beyer-Flores and Beverly Whipple

Satisfaction: The Art of the Female Orgasm by Cattrall, Kim and Mark Levinson

She Comes First: The Thinking Man's Guide to Pleasuring a Woman by Ian Kerner, Ph.D.

A New View of Women's Sexual Problems by Ellyn Kaschak and Leonore Tiefer

Satisfaction: The Art of the Female Orgasm by Kim Cattrall and Mark Levinson

Oral Sex He'll Never Forget by Sonia Borg, Ph.D.

Anal Pleasure & Health by Jack Morin Ph.D.

The Art of the Kama Sutra by Mallanaga Vatsyayana

Anatomy of Love: A Natural History of Mating, Marriage, and Why We Stray by Helen Fisher, Ph.D.

Any Man Can by Dr. Willian Hartman and Marilyn Fithian

California Exotics: www.calexotics.com

Taking a Closer Look at Basson's Model of the Sexual Response Cycle by Flannery, Joanne Z. Sexology International https://sexologyinternational.com/taking-a-closer-look-at-bassons-model-of-the-sexual-response-cycle

Confesiones de un Besologo by Ezequiel Lopez Peralta (Spanish)

HAPPY ENDING

A great and healthy relationship isn't about not having problems, difficulties, or differences. It is about staying deeply connected, understanding, accepting, supporting each other, and making love—enjoying a pleasurable sex life. In fact, there is no such thing as a problem-free individual or relationship. We all have a set of problems unique to us, but these sets of problems and virtues are different. When two individuals decide to be together and form a relationship, they are choosing not only each other, but their partner's problems as well.

A healthy relationship, then, is about two people willing to work and put effort into growing as individuals and as a couple by facing problems, difficulties, and differences in a constructive way through productive conversations, discipline, commitment, and actions. In that way, you can build up your relationship and strengthen your sex life to enjoy your love life fully. By building together a solid Three-Floor House, you and your partner can be happily connected and fulfilled through time as you age. Desire and intention are essential but, not enough to *make love 365 times a year*, effort and concrete actions are needed too.

Let's look back on how you have been constructing the path towards *making love 365 times a year* through the previous chapters. In Chapter 1, we discussed changing, building, and improving your sexual mindset. Challenging your sexual mindset can be the TOUGHEST part of learning about sexuality. As a child, many of us were fed with false beliefs and myths about sex. By updating and transforming your mindset about sexuality, you now know that sex is great for you, for your partner, and your relationship. You understand that you are a sexual being and will be until the end of your life. Remember, sexuality is who you are. Lovemaking is the expression of your love and who you are.

Nevertheless, a healthy sexual mindset—Sex Secret #1—while essential, is not enough to sustain a pleasurable sex life.

In Chapter 2, we discussed the importance of a healthy body and how being in a fair physical condition—the best you can—is necessary for active sex life. A healthy lifestyle covers everything from exercise and eating well to having a positive body image. All these changes may take time but are worth the effort! However, living a healthy lifestyle—Sex Secret #2—is still not enough.

The same is valid for loving feelings—Sex Secret #3—which are crucial, but not enough to sustain a pleasurable sex life. So, in Chapter 3, we discussed feelings and emotions, especially feelings towards your partner, and the LOVEX model to make love. We worked on communication in Chapter 4 and how many of us will avoid difficult and deep conversations—intimacy. You cannot *make love 365 times a year* without having these crucial conversations that are needed to get rid of resentment and build up emotional and sexual intimacy.

Being aware of feelings and how to express them correctly can be hard because we often refuse to talk to our partners about what is bothering us to "keep the peace." But now you know you must be open and honest with no fear! Expressions—Sex Secret #4—is vital to your relationship, in both verbal and non-verbal forms. Communication is well-known as the key to relationships, but by itself, it will not sustain a passionate love life.

Then, in Chapter 5, we learned a bit about pleasure—Sex Secret #5—and its significance for your overall well-being and a fulfilling love life. By now, you should recognize the importance of enjoying regular activities in your daily life, especially experiencing pleasure in sexual encounters. You should find more and more joy! Work on sexual pleasure and let go of yourself; you are ready for that! We are building "a stairway," and you should finish one step before moving to the next.

In Chapter 6, we explore eroticism—Sex Secret #6—which is the creativity part. You have already tackled the more difficult topics; therefore, it is time to open your imagination to create your "wild you" and so, your erotic self. Add your spice now, with "salsa y sabor" to make it hot…seduce, surrender, and conquer!

Finally, the fun part—Chapter 7—not meant to fix your relationship but to enhance it. Here you learn about sexual techniques—Sex Secret #7—for "playing" as much as you want with your partner. If you find yourself trapped in an unhappy or dysfunctional relationship, the worst thing you can do is to jump straight to the mechanics of sex to fix things between you and your partner. If you do so—jumping straight into sex—you will end up very disappointed and frustrated. Frustration is what happens to those couples in dysfunctional relationships when they try to fix their sex lives by getting kinky, taking pills, buying sex toys, or opening their relationship to solve their problems through sex; and missing all the rest.

Being erotic and kinky or being an expert on sexual techniques is not enough, either. It is the combination of these seven key elements—the 7 *Sex Secrets*—that make it happen, according to my professional and personal experience. By working together, you and your partner, one-by-one through these 7 *Sex Secrets*, you will be able to *make love 365 times a year*—and if it's not possible every day, there are plenty of days to cash in a raincheck—to build and maintain a passionate sex life.

Now that you and your partner have everything in place and have put together all the pieces of the puzzle, everything should be getting more comfortable and more fun. Lovemaking should always be an excellent experience for you— beyond orgasms—to connect in your own unique, intimate way. Together, you will find the closeness, the bliss, and the pleasure of two souls in love, and *in lust*, forever so you will be delighted! But, once again, every relationship needs to be cultivated, worked on, and updated; so, what better way to stay connected day-to-day but lovemaking? I know sometimes it isn't easy to do it; things happen, and we get crazy busy. But it can be much easier if you are determined, fearless, and have gratitude.

To end my book, I will share a dream I recently had. It was so bright that it seemed real for me, bringing me such a powerful feeling. And this was my dream: I dreamed of a chessboard folded that was in the living room of a small and beautiful mountain cabin. In a second scene, the chessboard appeared again, but down on the edge of a bed. The chessboard suddenly opened… it was red inside, made of fine wood with a symbol I couldn't recognize. Then words came from the chess board like a "revelation," saying: "Chess is for two people…you can have sex with many people, even great sex, in a threesome or foursome, in group sex, with a one-night stand or a hook-up, and so on, but you only make love with one person, the one you love. Because lovemaking ONLY happens between two people that deeply LOVE each other…" Then I woke up!

That is my simple message to you. Wake up, enjoy your love life, and *make love 365 times a year,* you can do it!

Thank you very much!

APPENDIX

The Lovemaking Wheel Questionnaire

This short questionnaire is about the *7 Sex Secrets*, the elements for vibrant sex life.

This questionnaire is about you; it doesn't matter if you are or aren't in a relationship, or if you are in a same-sex or opposite-sex relationship.

Please circle the answer that most relates to your present situation. If you don't have a partner, you can answer the seven questions with your "ex" in mind.

Circle only one answer:

1. **I believe sexuality is important for my overall wellbeing, and it is part of my lifestyle.**

   (1)　　(2)　　(3)　　(4)　　(5)

   Strongly　　　　　　　　　　**Strongly**
   Disagree　　　　　　　　　　**Agree**

2. **I have a healthy, energized body. I take proper care of it. I exercise regularly and eat heathy.**

   (1)　　(2)　　(3)　　(4)　　(5)

   Strongly　　　　　　　　　　**Strongly**
   Disagree　　　　　　　　　　**Agree**

3. I feel 100% happy, confident, safe, trustful, and full of positive feelings toward my partner.

(1)   (2)   (3)   (4)   (5)

Strongly   Strongly
Disagree   Agree

4. I freely express my thoughts and feelings. My partner and I have effective communication.

(1)   (2)   (3)   (4)   (5)

Strongly   Strongly
Disagree   Agree

5. I live my life with passion. Pleasure is important to me. I regularly experience pleasure in life.

(1)   (2)   (3)   (4)   (5)

Strongly   Strongly
Disagree   Agree

6. I feel sexy. Eroticism is part of my sexuality; it is within me. I enjoy my sexual self.

(1)   (2)   (3)   (4)   (5)

Strongly   Strongly
Disagree   Agree

7. **I am good in bed. I am confident and skillful when having sex. I know how to please.**

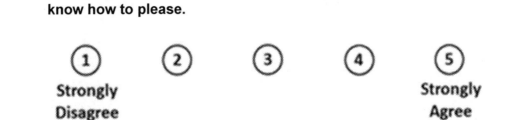

Now, take or transfer each answer or number to the Lovemaking Wheel, placing each number in its respective place, matching the respond number with the number in the Lovemaking Wheel. Then join the knots to make a wheel. This will be your Lovemaking Wheel!

Please, take the following Lovemaking Wheel and see how you and your partner are doing! You can find and download the questionnaire and the Lovemaking Wheel on the website.

The Lovemaking Wheel

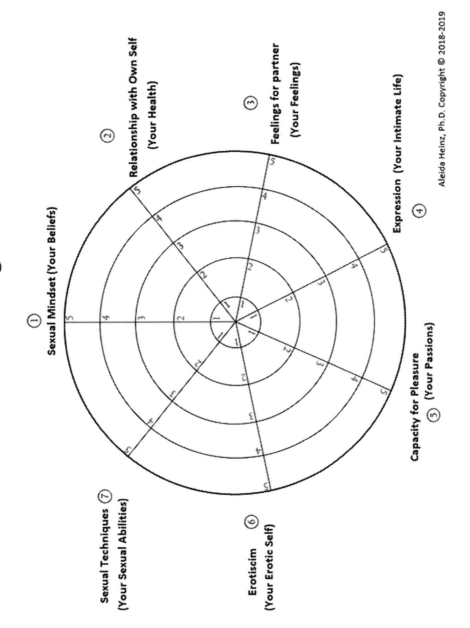

Sexual Mindset (Your Beliefs) ①

Relationship with Own Self ②
(Your Health)

Feelings for partner ③
(Your Feelings)

Expression (Your Intimate Life) ④

Capacity for Pleasure
⑤ (Your Passions)

Eroticiscim ⑥
(Your Erotic Self)

Sexual Techniques ⑦
(Your Sexual Abilities)

Printed in the United States
By Bookmasters

Statistics show that over sixty percent of married couples no longer have satisfying or even existent sexual relationships with their partners.

As a result, divorce, infidelity, loneliness, or couples living as roommates, or without sex, has become commonplace.

Make Love 365 Times a Year is an essential guide that can transform your relationship and your life by understanding what it takes to have a passionate love life. To unlock the potential to make love 365 times a year, you need energy, knowledge, intention, strategy, action—and most importantly—love.

Dr. Heinz, who has helped thousands of couples and people improve their love life, explores how to enjoy lovemaking. Learn how to:

- understand the difference between sex and lovemaking
- sustain a healthy and passionate love life over time
- stay connected with your partner while growing as an individual
- be ready for a better relationship
- understand love, lust, passion, and intimacy in long-term committed relationships

This book includes The Lovemaking Wheel, a chart the author created that serves to help you identify and evaluate your lovemaking behavior. Also, you will find unique models to better understand infidelity, relationships, eroticism, and pleasure.

Unlock *7 Sex Secrets* to enjoying a passionate love life and sustain a relationship filled with meaning with the lessons in this book.

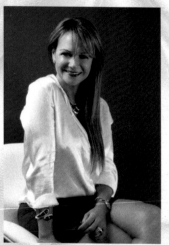

Aleida Heinz, PhD, is a lifetime board-certified sexologist, a PhD in human sexuality, a master's in sexology and couples counseling, and a Bachelor of Science in psychology and family science. She is one of the few experts who has successfully intertwined the fields of Couple and Sex Counseling to fully understand passionate relationships. Dr. Heinz has counseled couples and individuals from all around the world for more than 20 years. She operates a private practice in Charlotte, North Carolina and online, is happily married, has three adult children, and a dog.

www.aleidaheinz.com

U.S. $20.99

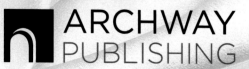
ARCHWAY PUBLISHING

ISBN 978-1-4808-9029-
5209
9 781480 890251